The doctor, the patient and the group

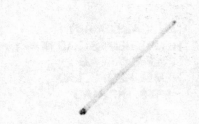

The doctor, the patient and the group

Balint revisited

Enid Balint, Michael Courtenay,
Andrew Elder, Sally Hull and Paul Julian

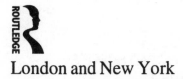

London and New York

First published in 1993
by Routledge
11 New Fetter Lane, London EC4P 4EE

Simultaneously published in the USA and Canada
by Routledge
29 West 35th Street, New York, NY 10001

© 1993 Enid Balint, Michael Courtenay, Andrew Elder, Sally Hull
and Paul Julian

Typeset in Times by LaserScript Limited, Mitcham, Surrey
Printed and bound in Great Britain by
Mackays of Chatham PLC, Chatham, Kent

A Tavistock/Routledge Publication

British Library Cataloguing in Publication Data

A catalogue record for this book is available from the British Library.

Library of Congress Cataloging in Publication Data

The Doctor, the patient, and the group: Balint revisited/by Enid
    Balint . . . [et al.].
    p. cm.
    Includes bibliographical references and index.
    1. Physician and patient – Congresses. 2. Physicians (General
    practice) – Congresses. 3. Medicine and psychology – Congresses.
    4. Balint, Michael – Congresses. I. Balint, Enid.
    [DNLM: 1. Physician–Patient Relations – congresses. 2. Physicians –
    psychology – congresses. 3. Psychoanalytic Therapy – methods –
    congresses. WM 460.6 D637]
    R727.3.D593   1992
    610.69′6 – dc20
    DNLM/DLC
    for Library of Congress   92-49166
                                                               CIP

ISBN 0–415–08052–5
    0–415–08053–3 (pbk)

Cases which are devoted from the first to scientific purposes and are treated accordingly suffer in their outcome; while the most successful cases are those in which one proceeds, as it were, without purpose in view, and asks oneself to be taken by surprises; . . . and always meets them with an open mind free from any presuppositions.

(Freud)

Contents

Preface

In the early 1950s, Michael Balint, whilst working at the Tavistock Clinic, decided to find out whether a psychoanalyst, who was also a doctor and had some experience of working with general practitioners, would be able to throw any light on some of the difficulties general practitioners were encountering at that time. The National Health Service had only just started and the status of general practice was low. Psychoanalysts were only beginning to enter the field of general medicine and were not yet accepted – in many places they still are not – as respectable members of the medical team. Balint thought that because general practitioners met all kinds of patients with all kinds of illnesses, many of whom had to be referred to specialists, they did not regard themselves as specialists at all. Many of them did not enjoy their work or know how to be comfortable in their role as general practitioners. The results of these ideas were first written down in a book called *The Doctor, his Patient and the Illness* (Balint 1957). Since then many books have been written, and many seminars have been held, all derived from his ideas and the ideas which have developed from them since. Balint's ideas, which sometimes still seem quite simple, proved to be far from simple when put into practice. There have been many changes, some creative, some less so, that have arisen whenever a Balint group meets. A constant and invigorating debate has occurred about what Balint groups are, or what they should be, and many different opinions continue to proliferate.

In this book we describe the ideas that developed out of a special group, which was suggested to one of us (E.B.) by Professor Marshall Marinker when he was Director of the MSD Foundation. Our aim was to examine developments that had occurred since the 1950s in order to determine what was still useful, what should be discarded, and what we had to offer which was new. We thought of it as a research project and during the years of working together (1984–7) we had no difficulty in discussing doctor–patient relationships, but we had more difficulty in discussing the theoretical developments or the usefulness of different ideas about research (see Chapter 8). We spent some time considering what research means, both in the medical field and outside it, particularly taking into account the discoveries of modern physicists, mathematicians and some of the assumptions made in other scientific environments. Many of these seemed to throw light on our endeavours to use and describe a method of research appropriate for studying the work of the general practitioner.

The idea that a psychoanalyst is necessary for this kind of enquiry has been questioned a great deal (Salinsky 1989). In reality few psychoanalysts work with general practitioners in this field now, and those that do vary very much in whether they wish to help general practitioners by telling them what they have learnt from their discoveries with patients who are in analysis or psychotherapy, or whether they wish to help the general practitioners by themselves learning about general practice and seeing how this makes sense to them.

In the 1990s, general practice seems to be changing fast. General practitioners have a new (1990) contract of employment and there are changes occurring that are likely to alter the structure of the National Health Service radically over the next few years. Nowadays new specialities have been created. There are now counsellors, for instance, some of whom work in general practice, as well as clinical psychologists and others. Many techniques are used by general practitioners to help them solve problems that are outside their ambit, and the pattern of these will vary from one doctor to another. Some would need a particular kind of specialist, whether a cardiologist or a counsellor, while others would feel competent in those fields themselves. This is a healthy state of affairs, but one which gives those of us who have worked in Balint groups a particular responsibility to examine the present situation and to demonstrate what cannot be passed on to others. This book will endeavour to show what is intrinsic to general practice: what general practitioners cannot avoid whether they want to or not, and whether this is helped by work in Balint groups. If psychoanalysts are involved in such work it is not their theory that helps but their ways of looking at patients and listening to them. From the very beginning Michael Balint pointed out that doctors do not need instruction – they get plenty of that in medical school and need it badly during their first few years of training – but they need something else afterwards, and that 'something else' is rather difficult to introduce, particularly to people who have been instructed for so many years. The something else is more than knowledge or facts. It cannot be taught; only discovered.

Perhaps the essence of Balint groups has always been to share experiences and enable people to observe and rethink aspects of their relationships with patients and their work as doctors. Medical schools could not be expected to teach them to do this, as first they have to teach them about the intricacies of modern medicine. One might call the medical school approach 'one-person' medicine. It would be too muddling and complicated for the student to learn about human relations, or 'two-person' medicine, when he was also having to learn about the diagnosis and treatment of either minor or severe body-centred illnesses.

This book sets out to describe Balint work as we see it now, in the 1990s, to emphasise the differences between this and previous ideas, and to answer some of the questions left unanswered in earlier books. We have chosen to illustrate our ideas by clinical example this time, and not by clinical histories. Clinical histories can be fascinating to read, but at the end of the history the reader can be left wondering where the theory and the practice fit together; we want to avoid that confusion. We have deliberately confined ourselves to a small number of illustrative cases, sometimes using the same patient to demonstrate different aspects of our ideas from chapter to chapter, hoping thereby to emphasise the many different angles from which a single case can be viewed. We wanted to find out how we might help patients in ordinary general practice contacts, but in a different way from the 'flash' phenomenon, as described in *Six Minutes for the Patient* (Balint & Norell 1973). We concentrated on observing how patients jerked us out of our usual rut, by one kind of surprise or another.

In a sense this book will be about 'Balint revisited' but it will also be concerned with the future of Balint work. We hope it will illustrate its essential nature, which is to add to the pleasure, satisfaction and competence of doctors in their ordinary work. The aim is not to teach a speciality, nor has it been so for a long time, but to leave these specialities to the specialists. The aim is to get to the heart of the matter with general practitioners whose burdens are great and whose satisfactions can sometimes be hidden because adequacy continues to be measured, by both general practitioners and patients, in terms formulated by specialists.

If patients feel that their doctors are inadequate it can be as much because the doctor himself is feeling inadequate, as the patient already feels so when he first approaches his doctor. It seems that general practitioners can feel inadequate because they are not specialists, but very few specialists feel inadequate because they are not general practitioners and therefore do not know how to work with patients who have no illness requiring specialist help. This is a strange state of affairs. The change in doctors after attending Balint groups might be defined as partly to do with enabling them to tolerate uneasiness and incoherence more comfortably – as well as enabling them to harness these uncomfortable feelings for the benefit of their patients.

Enid Balint, Ramsbury
1992

Acknowledgements

The work reported in this book was carried out in a seminar led by one of us (E.B.) which met at the MSD Foundation during university term-time between 1984 and 1987. It is based upon the case reports submitted by the general practitioner members of the research group. Apart from the authors these were: Dr James Carne, Dr Jane Dammers (until December 1986), Dr Marshall Marinker (until June 1986), Dr Jack Norell and Dr Lenka Speight.

A research group was suggested to Enid Balint by Marshall Marinker while he was Director of the MSD Foundation. The Foundation kindly paid a leader's fee to Enid Balint for the first two years of our work. It also made a room available for our weekly meetings, and provided recording equipment and photocopying facilities so that the seminars could be transcribed. These were usually typed commercially but at one time or another were also transcribed by Rosemary Courtenay and Christine Simpson to whom we are most grateful.

In 1985, Dr Martin Rossdale joined us to help with the scientific focus of our work. He stayed until the end of the weekly seminars in 1987.

We are grateful to the Balint Society who gave us a start-up grant. We are also particularly grateful to Dr Kaj Rasmussen of Denmark who awarded us a generous research grant in 1986. This donation allowed us to pay for the transcription of our seminars without which our work would not have gone forward.

We are indebted to our patients who are recounted here. To preserve their privacy we have substituted names, disguised their jobs and altered locations as well as the names of their doctors. These changes are consistent throughout the text so that the patients can be followed as they are described from different points of view in various chapters.

Lastly, we would like to express our thanks to the other group members who joined us on an exciting journey and entrusted to us the task of writing up the three years' work we undertook together.

EB, MC, AE, SH, PJ

Part I
Setting the scene

1   Next patient, please . . . .

> . . . it happens not so infrequently that the relationship between patient
> and doctor is strained, unhappy, or even unpleasant.
>
> (Balint 1957:11)

The first 'Balint book' (*The Doctor, his Patient and the Illness*) was a major
contribution to making sense of medicine, in the general practice field at any
rate, and its distilled findings have lived on. The 'apostolic function', the
'doctor as a drug', the 'collusion of anonymity', the 'unorganised illness' are
among the new jargon developed by the 'old guard'. But thirty years on is
the jargon understood, and is it still useful? The trouble with jargon is that it
takes on a life of its own and may become stifling to new growth.

Imagine yourself at the beginning of morning surgery. As the first
patient is called into the consulting room, do you consider for a moment
what you are expecting from the patient? Are you faintly aware of your
bio-availability at nine o'clock in the morning? Are you really prepared to
accept the coordinating responsibility in the care of your patient? Are the
hypotheses you generate in response to the patient's complaint allowed to
remain unorganised? Frankly, it is doubtful. If not, why should this be so?
Is it that damned apostolic function again, or is it that the change in
personality was insufficient? Or is it something not yet identified?

Let's go back to morning surgery again. You look at the list of your
appointments. The receptionists have booked you solid, and you have to
attend a trainer–trainee meeting at lunchtime. There's Mrs Bloggs who is
coming to see you for the second time this week with her usual manipulative
whingeing, there is Mr Briggs coming to have his hypertension monitored,
and Miss Bottomley is back, probably with her vaginal discharge again. Are
you sitting comfortably? Shall we begin? You have twenty-odd people to
see, a time constraint and a sinking feeling in the pit of your stomach. How
will you ration your charge of energy to cover the necessary personal
contacts you are going to make over the next two hours or so?

The likelihood is that you are going to put your mind into a well-worn and economical gear until such time that there seems to be a need for change, whatever that means. Is it rather like Newton's first law of motion: 'Every body remains in a state of rest or of uniform motion in a straight line, unless it is compelled by impressed forces to change that state'?

Let us consider the possible forces. First comes *novelty*. A new patient is always something of a challenge. Perhaps also a refreshment. A relief from chronic problems. The doctor brings an unbiased mind to the interview, unless something goes awry during the patient's contact with reception, or the doctor has negative feelings towards patients with green hair. The prospect of a new relationship can be stimulating, as it puts the general practitioner on a par with a specialist sitting in an outpatient clinic. Perhaps we enjoy returning to the hospital mode from the jungle of general practice.

Take the case of Mr F. He came urgently one evening, without an appointment, because he was over-breathing. A pre-clinical student was sitting in on the surgery, so there was pressure to relate the clinical picture to pre-clinical studies. The symptom was rapidly abolished by getting the patient to re-breathe the air from a brown paper bag, a splendid illustration to the student of the application of physiological principles. Mr F. is thirty-five, a thickset builder who smokes thirty cigarettes a day. He is in his second marriage to a wife a little older than himself, having three daughters, by his first wife, living with him. Although it was the first time doctor and patient had met, he had seen a female partner previously, who had noted that he had remarked that he had been 'considering the advantages of single life'. In the notes from his previous doctor it was seen that he had suffered from chest pains the previous year, and had been admitted to hospital to exclude a myocardial infarct. An infarct had not been confirmed, but it was clear that Mr F. thought he had had one when the illness was discussed in the current consultation.

It seemed likely that the confusion had arisen from the fact that the hospital doctor had said at the time of his discharge, 'You will get a heart attack if you continue to smoke thirty cigarettes a day'. The general practitioner offered to let him read the hospital report, but he declined. On further exchange there seemed to be an association between the over-breathing and returning home in the evening, as there had been several less severe attacks on his way home on previous days. It all pointed to domestic stress, but open-ended questions did not produce confirmation of this speculation. He was invited to think about what might have made him so anxious and to come the following week. He didn't come then, and in fact never saw the doctor again.

While on the face of it this was a clinical success in terms of symptom relief, the basis of the anxiety producing over-breathing remained obscure.

Did he feel humiliated by having made such a fuss when the treatment was so simple? Did he find it impossible to discuss problems with his marriage with a male doctor in the presence of a (female) student? Perhaps his mistaken idea about having had a heart attack had been useful to him in exciting sympathy and a protected lifestyle? The doctor had acted like a good detective, but had not gained the confidence of his patient. The hospital doctor approach had interfered with a general practice type of relationship. But the new relationship can be stimulating. The doctor has to get to know the new patient, as it is always said that it is the continuing relationship of general practitioners with their patients which is so valuable. Do we agree? Considering that there is roughly a twenty per cent turnover of patients in city areas, and that only about half the patients will have been on the doctor's list for more than five years in that setting, a large percentage of the practice population will not have been known for very long. The building up of a relationship is a process which needs the active participation of both patient and doctor, and this clearly depends upon what the doctor and the patient bring to the relationship. It may be built on a shallow basis, either because the doctor has unconscious prejudices, or because the patient wishes to play his cards very close to his chest!

Only if the patient has a consuming need to express distress will the doctor learn much about the patient quickly. In that event it will almost always lead to a greater understanding of the patient as a person in the course of the diagnostic process. However, in the absence of a circumstance leading to deeper understanding, a shallow, often collusive, relationship may develop in which the doctor thinks the patient is well known and understood. The pair come to a *modus vivendi* which apparently serves well for a time until the chips are down.

The second force may be a *surprise* occurring in the context of a long relationship. Take the case of Mrs Susan Towle, a woman in her late fifties who had been a patient of the doctor for thirty years. She came after being suddenly widowed, her husband having dropped dead in the street while they were out shopping together. He had suffered emphysema for years, but there had been no indication of impending disaster. As he had not attended any doctor in the practice for some time, he was a coroner's case. His wife had seen him after the post-mortem, and was deeply shocked at the way his cranium had been removed for examination of the brain and then stitched back. This had been immensely distressing to her, and there was an implied reproach that the post-mortem had not been obviated by the issue of a death certificate by the practice. She was obviously grieving deeply about her loss, which was somewhat surprising to the doctor as they had never been a close couple in his estimation. They had one daughter, who had been a baby when the doctor first met the family, and Mrs Towle had told him that there had been little in the way of sexual relations after the baby was born, as her husband had become disinterested. Mrs Towle had needed a good deal of attention medically over the years, as she suffered from bronchiectasis, and had recurrent depression as well. A rather bantering doctor–patient relationship had been established, with frequent dismissive remarks about family troubles and her own. Her daughter had had three children, each by different men. One of the children was severely asthmatic and so was often in need of support.

There had always been a feeling of warmth in the relationship with Mrs Towle, and she had often brought presents back for the doctor from where she went on holiday. She worked as a bus conductress, and was always amusing about the goings on at the bus garage, in terms of trade union and management issues. This time, however, the doctor was profoundly affected by her grief. He was also astounded by his absence of real understanding about the patient as a person over the years. Even though it had been clear that she dealt with painful issues by making something of a joke about them, the depth of feeling between her and her husband had not been appreciated. He had rarely attended the doctor in spite of his emphysema, and usually only when his wife bullied him into coming, which in retrospect might have given a clue about the nature of the relationship.

Knowing someone for a long time, or even knowing a family for a long time, may not reveal much in the way the individual or the family relate with one another. Length of time in a relationship is a different dimension from depth of understanding. Misconceptions can become ossified. There is the nasty possibility that general practitioners know very little about a lot of their patients, and this knowledge will have probably been gathered piecemeal in the course of a number of contacts over the years. Doctors may come to feel they know their patients better than they really do.

A third force for change is a *realisation* that over-identification has occurred. Mrs Angela Denton, a divorced woman of thirty-five, brought her elder son, Wayne, aged eleven, saying he seemed to be deaf (this case is reported in full in Part IV – The Booklet). The implication in her story was that he was not listening to what she said. The doctor discovered on examination that he had a genuine high-tone deafness, and while this obviously pleased Wayne, the doctor failed to notice the effect this had on his mother. The doctor had a clinical student sitting in with him, and as Mrs Denton rose to go she remarked to the student how wonderful the doctor was. The doctor immediately felt that this was a coded signal that he had rejected her distress by identifying with Wayne; and found himself only able to say that they should return for follow-up the following week.

When they did, Wayne was dismissed quickly as his hearing was improved with treatment for his catarrhal otitis, but Mrs Denton broke down in tears because she felt that the doctor thought she had been beastly to Wayne, which was then discussed.

A fourth force is the weight of *past knowledge* bearing on a new presentation. Miss Jean Carter, aged twenty, was the youngest of three children, having two older brothers. Her mother suffered from manic-depressive psychosis, and was maintained on lithium, but she had been close to suicide on occasion. Miss Carter came complaining of early waking and feeling generally low. She ascribed this to a change in her conditions at work. She used to work in a chatty office with lots of girls, but now she worked in a small room with a male workaholic, who was pleasant enough but hardly spoke to her. The doctor elicited depressive symptoms, but felt inhibited about relating them to those of her mother openly during the consultation. He was acutely aware of the possible similarity, but was unsure of the effect on Miss Carter, if she had not made a connection herself. At follow-up the next week she reported that she had slept better, but had had a nightmare. She had dreamed she had been in a car driving down a cul-de-sac and crashed into the wall at the end of the street. She had then been unable to get out of the car. She had woken up screaming, and was surprised she had not woken the household. She had said the previous week that she had felt like screaming when she was in the office, and the doctor reminded her of this. She was unconvinced by this association, saying she had been dealing with car-crash claims in the office. The doctor was then able to raise the question of her mother's health in terms of it being difficult to tolerate a depressed person in the house. However, it transpired that Miss Carter had left home a year previously, not on account of being unable to tolerate her mother, but because of her father nagging her about domestic chores while her mother was in hospital. She had stayed with a girlfriend until her recent return home. She had a steady boyfriend, though recently her sexual appetite had decreased. The doctor was then able to ask her if she was worried about becoming like her mother, but Miss Carter replied that this was not so, as her mother had been 'really ill'. She decided she wanted to return to work, and give the job a month's trial. In the event she had another office move, and her symptoms evaporated. The doctor felt he had hardly known the patient before, though she had been a patient all her life, and his knowledge of the family history may have distorted his judgement in relation to her symptoms.

What the doctor does know can obviously have a profound effect on the consultation. It can illuminate it sometimes, but can also affect it in a negative way. Returning to the scene where the general practitioner is about to begin a surgery, the names of the patients on his appointment list will close his mind as often, or perhaps more often, than they open it. It is as if the prospect of meeting the patient is a painful prospect. What is the nature of this pain?

Certainly, a fifth force is prejudice born of *the pain* of a long unsatisfactory relationship being suddenly overturned. Lawrence B., a man of sixty, having taken early retirement from the post office on account of chronic back trouble, had been a patient for thirty years. He was married to a woman some five years younger, who suffered from manic-depressive psychosis. They had two daughters. One was unmarried, but had a daughter, while the other was engaged. The family had been Jehovah's Witnesses for a long time, and the daughter with the illegitimate child had been expelled on that account. Both daughters currently shared a flat some way from the parental home. Their mother spent a good deal of time visiting them, and this was a source of marital conflict. A long time ago there had been sexual difficulties between Mr and Mrs B., and in the course of trying to deal with this, it emerged that homosexual feelings were expressed by Mr B., though couched in somewhat religious imagery. This had made the doctor uncomfortable at the time and the work did not prosper, so that neither the marital relationship nor the poor work-record improved, and eventually the patient drifted into seeing another partner in the practice.

However, the doctor had recently been called to Lawrence's house where he was lying in bed, with a normal pulse and temperature, and without any physical signs, though he had obviously been suffering from a virus illness for some days. The doctor was dismissive and told the patient to continue taking the cough mixture he had bought. There was a feeling in the doctor that he had invested quite a lot of time and energy in treating Lawrence in the past, usually without success, and was unwilling to do so again. A few days later Lawrence came to the surgery looking really ill, accompanied by his wife, and was found to have signs of consolidation at the right base. He was prescribed antibiotics and a follow-up arranged.

It dawned on the doctor what he had and had not been doing. The doctor–patient relationship was burnt out, but the patient had nevertheless been able to send out signals of distress when he came to the surgery, having persevered in keeping in contact with the doctor who had visited him, in spite of having deteriorated. The fifth force may be described as the patient hitting the doctor over the head!

A little while later Lawrence made an appointment to see the doctor again. The doctor was surprised that he had not gone to see one of his partners, after what might well have appeared as second-class care for the acute respiratory infection, and his curiosity was awakened. This time the patient did not even complain of back trouble, which had continued as the theme for visits to the practice over the years, but of feeling low spirited. It emerged that the back trouble had occasioned early retirement, and he was now generally at a loose end. He did not want to stay at home all day, as his wife was busy shopping and doing the housework, and visiting her sick mother every other day. The breakdown of the engagement of his elder daughter had also made him unhappy. The doctor considered he was depressed, and arranged to see him regularly.

On one occasion he brought a present in the form of an illustrated book produced by the Jehovah's Witnesses to interest unbelievers in their message. The illustrations were bright, stylised pictures of a Garden of Eden kind of existence, peopled by nubile young people, and it was obvious that the patient eagerly awaited the transformation of his present drab world into this blissful kind of existence. There was even a hint of trying to evangelise the doctor, who reflected his perception of the situation back to the patient with an apparently positive response.

A few days later, while doing some quick shopping one afternoon, the doctor happened to see Lawrence sitting rather disconsolately on a bench in the middle of a pedestrian shopping precinct. The doctor didn't approach him directly at that moment, but used the observation during the next consultation, and offered anti-depressant medication, which he declined. This seemed connected with his wife being on long-term medication of this kind, and he felt he was not ill enough to merit it, and also that she would know what he was taking. It would be a symptom of failure in his religious faith.

He continued to attend the doctor for some time and appeared to improve. However, some time later it was noticed he was seeing another partner again, although he did come once more, complaining of his back. But the doctor no longer felt rejective towards him, as a permanent change in the relationship had occurred.

These cases illustrate the kind of forces which may cause a change in the doctor's clinical conduct of a case. The question they raise is why general practitioners feel comfortable to continue 'in a straight line' in the absence of such powerful forces.

The usual mode of working might be likened to the drive notch on an automatic gearbox of a car. If all seems to go smoothly the doctor takes no unusual action. If there seems to be a difficulty he may shift the selector to lock either second or even first gear. In dire emergencies he may even use a kick-down change to negotiate what appears as a hairpin bend on a mountain pass! The question is how much perceived labouring of the doctor's engine is required to make him alter the setting? Is it that change is only considered if he finds himself in the position of an automatic gearbox hunting for the right gear as the incline steepens?

Perhaps we still live in the grip of the myth that general practitioners know their patients well. In reality we only know what patients want us to know. This is quite appropriate. We are not in the business of uncovering secrets for the sake of full information. Our knowledge of the patient may range widely, but still remain shallow, until such time that there is a need for a closer doctor–patient relationship, perhaps associated with a crisis for the patient. Then our knowledge may go deep over a small part of the total spectrum. We should not feel badly about this – the patients are using us as professionals. There is a much greater danger if the myth drives us into the position of saying, concerning the material of the doctor–patient relationship: 'never mind the quality, feel the width'. If we wait upon our patients' needs it will not only ease our burden, but stimulate a new vista of interest.

NOTE

Several of the chapters which follow contain transcriptions of discussions. The conventions used in transcribing are described on p. 106.

2 Whatever happened to Balint?

I have mentioned that in Utopia the specialist will not be a superior mentor, but the general practitioner's expert assistant. Conversely, this means that the general practitioner will no longer be able to disappear behind the strong and impenetrable facade of a bored, overworked, but not very responsible dispenser of drugs and writer of innumerable letters, certificates and requests for examinations; instead he will have to shoulder the privilege of undivided responsibility for people's health and well-being, and partly also for their future happiness.

(Balint 1957:289)

At the centre of medicine there is always a human relationship between a patient and a doctor. This is the unchanging core of medical work, despite whatever technical advances are made. We can read *Hamlet* or any great work of literature from the past, and learn a lot about human life, despite the circumstances of Hamlet's life being radically different from our own. Similarly, in the lives of past doctors we can discern the same core ingredients of a medical life that any modern doctor will recognise despite the immense differences in the medical means at his disposal. The clothing of medicine is constantly changing; the core of medicine changes little.

Why is this central area of our work so hard to study? And why has it been relatively neglected in recent general practice research, particularly since in general practice it is closer to the essence of the subject than it is in other branches of medicine?

No two consultations are ever the same. If a quite straightforward 'case' is presented separately to two doctors in role play, the resulting consultations are usually quite different. Doctors are as variable as their patients. In any morning surgery there are many different directions a doctor might take with his patients. Even at the level of making traditional medical diagnoses the choice is likely to be wide. Making diagnoses, although important, is only a small part of a doctor's work. A lot else occurs alongside.

Take the case of Arthur Jennings. He presented to his doctor as a dapper looking man of sixty-five, although his actual age was eighty! He had first consulted her four years previously with miscellaneous aches and pains which had been diagnosed as polymyalgia. He had refused a temporal artery biopsy in hospital because that would have meant leaving his wife alone at home. He had been started on corticosteroids and seen regularly every month or two for a check-up and an ESR. He always wore an old grey suit and a flat cloth cap lined carefully with tissue paper. The doctor felt she didn't know him well, but had discovered he had a daughter living quite close by, and that his wife, suffering from dementia, was under the care of an older partner. At his most recent follow-up, the doctor asked after his wife, and was told that she had just died. Only then did the doctor notice he was wearing a black suit. He talked for about a quarter of an hour about the distress he felt at the death of his wife. He had been shocked by the way the ambulance men had carried this overweight woman down the stairs with her legs dangling over the edge of the stretcher. The hospital had called later to let him know that she had died. The doctor felt badly. How could she not have known what had been going on? She feared for him in the future, now alone and relieved of his deeply caring role. What had his wife's hospitalisation meant to him? He had not accompanied her apparently, and this seemed, somehow, out of character.

Two months later he came in without having made an appointment, complaining of neck pain. There was nothing significant to find on examination of his neck. The doctor said, 'It's painful to be alone'. He laughed this off. He then shared his distress with the doctor over some black-rimmed cards sent by the undertakers, 'an awful reminder, they shouldn't have done it'. The doctor remarked that it was a good thing that this neck pain had not happened when he was looking after his wife and he agreed. The doctor had difficulty in remembering this when she came to report the follow-up, and also noticed that she had made no written note on the last two consultations, suggesting that her feelings had altered her usual style.

This fragment of a case demonstrates the intertwining themes of orthodox clinical medicine and a human relationship in the context of professional work. Whether a 'unified field theory'[1] can be applied in such a case is a matter of debate, but in practical terms an understanding and timely consideration of both the somatic and emotional strands appears to have satisfied both patient and doctor sufficiently. This is typical general practice. How are we to study and evaluate such work?

It has been well established that experienced general practitioners watching the same video recordings of consultations vary considerably when invited to attach diagnoses or evaluate the consultations observed (Jenkins &

Shepherd 1983:403). After all, in the snapshot of Mr Jennings and his doctor, even sticking to conventional diagnostic lines there would be a choice of at least polymyalgia, cervical spondylosis, anxiety or reactive depression. Medical diagnoses make very limited descriptions of general practice consultations. To widen the picture, something more could be added about the patient's expectations of a visit to the doctor, perhaps something of his past, or fears for the future, his relationships with other people and himself, and something of his past patterns of reaction and capacity for change. This enlarges the portrait and might also include any clues the patient gives about why he is coming to the doctor at the present time. We would then be nearer a whole-person diagnosis, more suitable for general practice, but the scene is still entirely patient-centred. The doctor is nowhere yet in view. The importance of this omission, and the severity of the error it induces, increase the more the patient's personal life and feelings are taken into account. The doctor and patient are influencing each other all the time, and cannot be considered separately. This is analogous to Winnicott's idea 'where there is an infant there is also a mother' (Winnicott 1972). Thus where there is a patient there is also a doctor.

Today's patient may seem different tomorrow and the same patient would be seen differently on the same day by different doctors. Not only would the patient be seen differently, but he would be behaving and presenting differently. Patients learn how their doctors like them to behave and what sorts of illness to have, whilst doctors have their own interests, strengths and hobbyhorses, and encourage patients along these lines. The one cannot be considered without the other. Both are constantly influenced by what each can bear. After all, they are not often trivial matters that bring the two together. The patient must somehow be helped to continue life in his own way, and the doctor must be able to carry on his work sufficiently at ease with himself and all the other demands he has to meet. It is the study of this complex phenomenon, the dialogue between a doctor and a patient each affecting the other, that is the true study of the doctor–patient relationship.

After bringing the doctor into view our canvas is nearly complete. However, it still needs to be remembered that much of what we have included is constantly changing; nothing is static; that the doctor only has scattered 'six minute' views of any of this; that in many cases the doctor would also be seeing other members of the same family; that in general practice there are often personal relationships tied up with work, patients who have become friends, friends who have become patients, people known in the community and so on; to say nothing of the effect that off-stage characters, like a previous difficult or disturbed patient, may have on the next consultation or two down the line; or the doctor's relationship with his partners and the effect of patients criss-crossing between them; and of course, somewhere just out of view, there is the larger world, with its values and pressures, and the doctor's personal life.

By describing the landscape of general practice in this way, we have made it seem more orderly than it is! The truth is more chaotic. All these factors play their part simultaneously, in no particular order and with varying importance at different times. Our field is both massive and intricate, a vast area without easily discernible patterns or shape; too much to take in.

The glare from this has a blinding effect when we try to study the subject. We are confused and quickly turn away or shield our eyes. This phenomenon occurs both at the individual level, when a doctor is faced with a patient, and also when as general practitioners we set out to research our subject. In the consulting room it leads typically to a doctor focusing on what is familiar, or concentrating on only a small part of the patient's presentation. Academically, it could be argued that the same phenomenon has had a marked influence on the development of general practice research. When we attempt to bring the subject into sufficient focus for research purposes, we tend to turn for help to what is available to us from our medical past or to disciplines other than our own; different sets of spectacles that enable us to focus on one small part of the landscape at a time, epidemiological ones, cardiological ones, sociological ones and so on. The list could be long. Marshall Marinker in an editorial entitled 'Journey to the interior: the search for academic general practice' (Marinker 1987) fears 'for academic general practice that it may develop along lines laid down by fashionable research which is neither *consonant* with the clinical experience of general practitioners nor *central to their concerns*'. General practice research often seems to present the working doctor with different imported views of his work from which the basic feel of his territory is hardly recognisable. It does not seem to bear enough relevance to the problems thrown up by daily clinical practice. What has been difficult to find is a more authentic view, an approach to research that brings into focus the characteristic challenges of consulting in the surgery.

Facilitating the observation of work in general practice, and evaluating it, has always been one of the main aims of the Balint methodology. The Balint group is designed to include interpersonal variables amongst the data observed in what has always been a part training, part research venture. In this way it gets closer to the feelings of daily clinical practice and pays particular attention to personal factors, which are easily overlooked, and which considerably influence how useful doctors are to their patients. Balint groups not only include these important factors within their field but also enable relevant observation of them. In this respect they differ from the many other forms of small group work which are now common in medical education. Whilst commenting on a recent Balint book, *While I'm Here, Doctor* (Elder & Samuel 1987), Freeling says that it should be read 'because it affords descriptions of what characterises general practice as a discrete discipline' (Freeling 1988:1122). Conrad Harris in a lecture on general practice research mentions 'the only truly ethnographic research method that general practice has evolved – the Balint group' (Harris 1989:315).

The traditional tendency in medical research has been to remove most of the complex variables of clinical work and leave only a tiny remainder for study, about which the researcher feels he can be 'objective'. Unfortunately, in general practice, what gets left out may have more bearing on the outcome than what gets left in! Just as in the measurement of relative motion a truer account is given if the speeds and directions of both subject and object are included, so it is in medical practice, where all the interactions of doctors and patients are relative to each other. Only by incorporating an understanding of the observer as well as the observed and the relative influence each has on the other can more accurate observations be made. If we are serious about whole-person medicine, or if audit is to progress to more than counting prescriptions or referrals to hospital, then our field of study must be long term and include both the patient and the doctor within its view.

Let us now go back to Mr Jennings. Four months later the doctor reported another follow-up. Mr Jennings had been the first appointment of the morning, and had remarked on what a lovely spring morning it was. He had been up since six o'clock watching the sunrise, and then went on to talk of climbing mountains during his war service. He was complimentary about the doctor's room and asked about her typewriter. 'Do you use that thing?' After five minutes or so the doctor felt she ought to begin the business part of the consultation and asked how he was. He seemed physically well and the doctor suggested a reduction in his dose of steroids, with which he agreed. He then went on to say he had an awful row with one of his daughters with whom he had very little contact – only one perfunctory phone call since his wife had died. He disapproved of her lifestyle and the man she lives with. He went on to say that he thought about his wife and his daughter quite a lot, but did not elaborate further, and the doctor felt unable to enquire further.

Eight months later, after the doctor had returned from maternity leave, he was her very first patient. He came in saying 'Where have you been then?' He complained that his aches and pains had worsened during her absence; for despite having seen her locum twice, who had reduced his steroids drastically, he had not discussed his symptoms. At the next follow-up a month later, he had stopped the small residual dose of steroids completely, on his own initiative. However, he complained of various aches and pains. His ESR was twenty-two. The doctor had prescribed some naproxen for him at their last contact, and this had eased his neck symptoms, but she now also restarted his steroids. The doctor opened up the discussion by asking what he was doing. He had sent a birthday card to his grandson, aged thirteen. His daughter had phoned and asked how he was, but told him not to discuss another grandson's divorce. 'I don't give much away' was his parting remark.

As this case develops, it is clear that there has been a considerable change in the way Mr Jennings and his doctor relate to each other. Before the death of his wife and the consultation in which the doctor was shocked into catching up with Mr Jennings's new situation (in which she also suddenly saw how little she had previously known about him), there was an almost unnoticed relationship, semi-ritual, with ESRs, adjustments of the steroid dose, and a minimal exchange of information between the two. Mr Jennings was seen as an elderly man with a 'flat cloth cap lined carefully with tissue paper'. Afterwards the picture changes. The patient's needs are different. The doctor has been alerted. Her task now is to keep her mode of medicine sensitive to whatever develops. She must still respect the patient's privacy but now they can share that understanding of his character, 'I don't give much away'. Mr Jennings now says things like 'Where have you been then?' and looks around admiringly enjoying the doctor's room and is reminded of his younger days climbing mountains! A very different Mr Jennings.

It is clear that the observation of the many strands in such a case is highly complicated. In discussing these follow-up reports, the group discussed many questions.

How much of the initial reserve when Mr Jennings mentioned that he often thought about his wife and daughter came from him or from the doctor? How much of Mr Jennings's changed state is due to his new relationship with his doctor? How much does the way this relationship develops tell us about Mr Jennings's other relationships, perhaps with his daughters and with his wife? It is clear that Mr Jennings likes his doctor. Has this always been so or have his feelings changed since the death of his wife, or is it only since then that the doctor has noticed that he likes her? How much of any of this is the doctor able to observe, and does it benefit the patient? How much of the doctor's initial sense of shock about not knowing more about Mr Jennings's wife was a just reaction or a feeling of guilt picked up from the patient? If the doctor misinterprets her reaction, does she then run the risk of trying to find out more than the patient wants her to know in the future? Pace is all important. The doctor and patient work this out together. What made the doctor stop the consultation after the first seven minutes and introduce what she saw as 'the business'? How are all these factors related to the variations in Mr Jennings's symptoms, and the doctor's varying reaction to those symptoms, sometimes altering the dosage of steroids, sometimes trying to relate them to his feelings of grief? To what extent are his symptoms a necessary part of his continuing contact with the doctor?

The doctor–patient relationship is the connecting thread that runs through all our work with patients. The focus of attention in general practice needs to include this relationship as well as all the various medical activities that it carries. In general practice the balance between these two is especially important and easily lost. It could be argued that attention to this balance is one of the key ingredients of general practice, and that if successful, it goes a long way towards determining the effectiveness of all the more specialised help patients get from ourselves and other sources.

Much of the work of general practice seems at first sight to overlap with that of other disciplines. It might appear that general practice is a little bit of a lot of different specialities all joined up. Even the way that vocational training is organised suggests this – a bit of paediatrics, geriatrics, gynae-cology and psychiatry, say, all mixed in the right proportions. Although it is true that general practice requires a good working knowledge of many subjects, any general practitioner will consider that such a description leaves out a lot of what gives the job its distinctive feel.

A thoracic surgeon, say, has a clearly defined anatomical area that concerns him, and associated expertise. There are aspects of his work that he has in common with other specialities but there is a definite core to his subject which is distinct. In the physiognomy of general practice, the most distinctive features can be difficult to discern. The general practitioner's basic position in the organisation of medical care is well enough known – accessible as a first port of call, custodian of continuity, and basic gate-keeper to the specialist services – but how can he best contribute in a way that others cannot? What is the general practitioner's particular expertise?

It is the unfortunate fate of generalists that everyone else seems to have a clear idea of how they should be spending their time. From so many more specialised viewpoints, the general practitioner's territory looks inviting. 'The GP is ideally placed . . . ' has become an almost ubiquitous phrase in the medical literature. With its own main characteristics poorly defined, the face of general practice becomes common ground for all who pass to etch out a reflection of their own particular interests. It is a fashionable view about almost everything, you name it . . . and 'the GP is ideally placed!'

The phrase usually ends an article by someone with a special interest, perhaps in alcoholism, drug dependency, diabetes or depression, in which they have scanned the vast untreated 'pathology' in the community and conclude, of course, that 'the GP is ideally placed . . . '. For the modern general practitioner there is an almost endless list of responsibilities and problems for which the doctor or a member of 'the team' is the prescription.

Whilst to a large extent the mass of general practitioners must quake or feel irritation as these suggestions roll in from people who are unlikely ever to have to sit in the general practitioner's hot seat, we do also seem strangely prone to inflict them on ourselves! If there is something particularly difficult to recognise about the general practitioner's own expertise, then sadly it would seem that we do not easily recognise it ourselves either!

The position is a little like that of a general gardener who has responsibility for the overall design of a great garden but instead of gaining satisfaction from his position, he overlooks it almost entirely and apologises for not being an alpinist or rose grower. It is perhaps worth enquiring why this phenomenon should be so pronounced amongst general practitioners. It should be clear that the specialist growers cannot bring their talents to the fore without the general gardener performing his function well. And to fulfil his own role best he will need to exercise a disciplined restraint, holding his attention on the overall design, not rushing too soon into too great a detail thereby losing his perspective, but waiting for the pattern and ways in which each of the various sections of the garden affect each other to emerge. Why is this so hard?

At the heart of our work lies a paradox. There are problems of definition. The most characteristic aspects of general practice work are intrinsically hard to define. It is not simply that our work is made up of little bits of everything (gynaecology, cardiology, etc). Rather, its essence lies in being an accessible generalist and in resisting such sets of definitions. It holds back from organising its focus too soon, in order that a deeper personal perspective may emerge which will enable connections to be made between different parts in the overall narrative of the patient's distress. It may be that the general practitioner is not ideally placed to be a mini-specialist in everything, but perhaps is ideally placed to gain some understanding of patients as people and use this for the benefit of their medical care. The Balint approach is a method of studying this; for studying how the doctor and patient relate, and through this central focus, examining how useful all the different facets of medical work are to both the patient and the doctor.

Balint work is frequently referred to in the present literature of general practice. There are many articles written describing, say, the attachment of a counsellor, a community psychiatric nurse or a psychotherapist in the general practice setting and the Balints' work is likely to be amongst the references setting the scene in the introductory section of the article. Important though the work of such attachments is, it is different from the lead the Balints gave to general practitioners to respect and study their own work with patients. A journey through the recent literature on the subject of emotional problems and general practice reveals some exceptional papers. For example, in 'Intimacy and terminal care' (Gilley 1988) the author illustrates, through a description of four cases, how the quality of the previous sexual relationship in a marriage and the capacity for the physical expression of intimacy can profoundly influence choices in terminal care and the quality of dying, when they are sensitively observed in the doctor–patient relationship and used for the patient's benefit. More representative of recent trends, however, might be 'Can general practitioners counsel?' (Rowland, Irving & Maynard 1989). None of the authors are general practitioners, and no cases are described. Balint work is referred to 'since Balint . . . general practitioners have been aware that patients can be helped by the use of counselling techniques', and the paper then goes on to define the impracticability of the general practice setting for what the authors call 'counselling' as defined by the British Association of Counselling. It does this in terms of the lack of time and specific training and the presence of one or two other 'non-counselling' expectations that patients might have of doctors! It concludes that 'it is essential to move beyond "practitioner flair" to guarantee reliable standards of care . . . through the benefits of counsellor attachment schemes'. This paper seems to miss the point that an understanding of the patient's emotional conflict, and how these are related both to the patient's illness and to the relationship between the patient and the doctor, isn't anything to do with 'counselling' but has everything to do with good medicine. That this aspect of being a good doctor is often called 'counselling' simply adds to the confusion. In 'Let's do away with counselling' (Harris 1987), the author puts the problem well. He attempts to show how 'by simply saying what we mean in plain English we . . . manage without counselling (the word) very well . . . and our patients will benefit by our precision'. He also describes how in the 1970s 'counselling' put down roots in ground previously cultivated by two separate traditions. 'One was the Balint approach, which tried to make general practitioners aware of the importance of the doctor–patient relationship in their handling of patients' emotional problems; the other was the movement for attaching social workers to general practice. They reflect (he says) a constant dilemma in general practice: whether we should learn to use new techniques ourselves or be content to recognise and refer.' He might have added that to scrutinise those very decisions is part and parcel of the Balint method.

If it is true that there are few studies by general practitioners taking the doctor–patient relationship as a principal focus, why is this? Why should this be so? It may be the case that general practitioners prefer the doing to the describing, or that it is thought perhaps a bit unBritish or unhealthy to look too closely at such things. As has already been described, part of the answer may lie in the considerable difficulty of looking at what goes on between doctors and patients in general practice, which must include observation of the doctor's part in this. How comfortable is this? The burdens and responsibilities of the consulting room are great and doctors often seem either apologetic or in pain over their work with patients. They may fear that looking will make things worse. Often the opposite is the case.

As doctors we are profoundly programmed towards action: actively pursuing diagnoses or the causes of whatever is troubling our patients and just as profoundly programmed towards active treatment. It is commonly thought that Balint work lays an additional load on the doctor's existing responsibilities for treatment, whereas it is more concerned with making observations. If it becomes assumed that an interest in Balint work implies some kind of added treatment responsibility for all the emotional problems amongst the doctor's list of patients, then it is hardly surprising that general practitioners might not want to know!

The prevailing view about Balint amongst many general practitioners might be that his contribution to the development of general practice was an important one but that it now belongs to history – it has been superseded and is no longer relevant. Consultation analysis, counsellor attachment schemes, the teaching of family interview methods, and holistic medicine have taken its place. Views as to what that contribution mainly consisted of would vary. In the main they would include something to do with discovering the importance and frequency of psychological factors in determining patients' symptoms, and the clues through which these are often presented to general practitioners. Balint work is often, quite erroneously, described as one of the items on a sort of medical menu from which the doctor is invited to select a suitable method or strategy for managing the problems that patients present.

It would seem that this view, that 'Balint is history', is partly true and partly false. It is perhaps one of the problems of a body of work being eponymously identified that it gives rise to a confusion between the work and the person. Clearly, quite a large part of Michael Balint's personal influence on the development of general practice does belong to the study of history. This would include a description of the particular context of British general practice in the 1950s and the difficulties it faced, Balint's own background as the son of a general practitioner, his life-long interest in medicine, and the early development of his (and his wife Enid's) ideas about how psychoanalysis could be helpful to doctors. It would include an account of the influence of these ideas on modern training for general practice and on the aims embodied in the foundation of the Royal College of General Practitioners. This is, of course, quite different from saying that the work itself, the method of studying general practice that the Balints developed, is no longer relevant or no longer has validity and vitality for present-day general practitioners. In any scientific enquiry all conclusions are provisional and need constantly re-examining in the light of further study. Similarly, the instrument itself which enables the observations to be made, the method, will only stand until a more sensitive one is developed. Certainly, some of the conclusions and findings of the earlier Balint work have become mummified and should be thought of as history, or at least re-examined. But the basic approach, the particular group method, the spirit of genuine enquiry, respect for the general practitioner's own attempts to help his patients, and the centrality of the doctor–patient relationship as the focus of study, all still have much to offer us. We would be very unwise to continue failing to make the distinction between what is dead in the Balint tradition and what is living.

Closely connected to the view that 'Balint is history' is the idea that knowledge proceeds progressively; that one development leads to another in a stepwise fashion; that once something is discovered, an orderly advance can be made by building on it. This is rarely true even in the evolution of our knowledge of the physical world, but is even less true of any understanding acquired about ourselves, which always has a tendency to be corrupted or lost. Balint work seeks to help doctors gain insight into the nature of their professional work and is therefore heir to these factors in the same way. In a sense every doctor, and certainly each new generation of doctors, has to discover afresh whatever there is to be learnt through the Balint method. It is a different kind of learning than the progressive acquisition of intellectual knowledge, and therefore needs constant renewal, and the need for this cannot become outdated.

NOTE

1 A theory sought by modern physicists which would successfully combine quantum mechanics with relativity theory.

3   Meeting points

> Thus the research could be conducted only by general practitioners
> while doing their everyday work, undisturbed and unhampered,
> sovereign masters of their own surgeries . . . (but) the doctors tried hard
> to entice the psychiatrists into a teacher pupil relationship . . .
>
> (Balint 1957:3)

The impetus which led to the first Balint groups sprang from two sources.
One was the courage of the general practitioners of the period who were
dissatisfied with things as they were; the other was a psychoanalyst,
Michael Balint, who was prepared to shed his usual setting and explore the
world of general practice. In doing so, they moved beyond the established
body of theory of both disciplines.

From early on, it was recognised that to incorporate psychoanalytic
theory or traditional psychotherapeutic skills into the fleeting pragmatic
encounters of the general practitioner's surgery was inappropriate. Over
time this way of working has drawn around it new ways of thinking about
interpersonal encounters, which are influenced both by psychoanalysis and
by general practice, but not bound by either. This chapter will attempt to
describe the contributions of each discipline to what becomes the focus of
attention in a Balint group.

Probably most doctors who have considered joining a group will bring a
number of assumptions about the nature of the work. They may assume that
only psychiatric cases are discussed, or that there are techniques to be
learned for gaining information or interpreting events in a patient's life.
There are likely to be preconceptions about how the group might think,
about what use the group makes of ideas from the psychoanalytic tradition
(especially if the leader happens to be an analyst). Many of these themes
will never surface explicitly during the working life of the group, and so
may be the cause of disappointment, or at least of puzzlement and mis-
understanding. This is not to say that general practitioners who work in

Balint groups need to have any theoretical knowledge about psycho-analysis. Indeed, an anxiety about 'knowing things' is counterproductive and prevents an attitude of spontaneous thought in the group, just as an anxiety about having an appropriate knowledge base in general medicine may prevent a doctor listening attentively to the patient. Analysts and general practitioners alike contribute observations which are determined by their own professional training. As they work together a group identity develops, and the leader and the members mutually influence each other's views of the case material. It is in the setting of this group 'laboratory' that new observations can be made about doctors and their patients, and change can occur.

ENCOUNTER AND MUTUALITY

Most of the everyday work of general practice is carried out at the inter-personal level, rather than dealing with intra-psychic phenomena which are largely the world of the psychoanalyst. What the patients say and do is largely taken at face-value, and responded to in a pragmatic, straight-forward way. Alongside this commonsensical general practice view lie aspects that are sought out in the work of Balint groups and are derived from the psychoanalytic tradition; a concentration on the emotions aroused by the encounter, and the inclusion of the doctor within the field of view. It is accepted that clinical observation, emotional response, and the gaining and giving of therapeutic satisfaction are all mutual processes. The import-ance of a personal encounter with the patient and the mutuality of that process is intuitively understood by all good doctors. One of the main ways in which a patient in distress can begin to feel better is by being within a relationship which itself can promote healing or change. This may not necessarily be one in which a lot of explanatory work is done; just as often it will be a relationship in which there is simply a recognition and accept-ance of the distress which the patient offers, and which is felt by the doctor.

Recognising the central importance of two-person psychology within general practice may explain the stress that is placed on the doctor–patient relationship, and why work within the group focuses on this aspect, attempting not to stray too far towards the area inhabited exclusively by the patient or, as can happen, into the personal or intra-psychic world of the doctor.

The case of Mr Arthur Jennings (first reported in Chapter 2) illustrates this. A woman doctor sees a dapper elderly man of eighty. She has been seeing him regularly to monitor his polymyalgia, for which he takes steroids. He is reticent, and she knows little about him except that he cares for his wife who has dementia. One day it crosses her mind that the wife will eventually die. She asks after her, and the patient says that she died recently. The doctor then notices the patient's black suit. He tells her of the anguish he felt, and how degrading it was for his wife to be carried out on a stretcher with her feet hanging over the edge and banging against the wall. She died in hospital within twenty-four hours.

Over the next few months there were several consultations, in part concerned with alterations to the steroid dose, but which also involved the doctor being available to hear what was happening to the patient. For this patient that level of involvement was sufficient, and when the doctor attempted to be more explicit about what was happening it didn't seem to help. For example, on one occasion when he arrived for an urgent appointment with some neck pain which was unrelated to his polymyalgia, the doctor suggested that it must be painful having to live alone, but this idea was shrugged off.

This patient appeared to want his doctor to be attentively present, not to be interpretive, and given that sort of relationship he could continue to come and talk about things at his own pace. To do this effectively the doctor needs to make continual observations on the process and content of the doctor–patient relationship, and make informed decisions about how to intervene, or when not to intervene.

Another aspect of mutuality and personal involvement is illustrated by the work that occurred within the group after the presentation of this case. In order to be able to attend properly to what the patient brings, the doctor needs to allow himself to identify with the patient. This involves letting himself be drawn into the emotional life of the patient, to stand alongside him, to empathise with him. But having once allowed this identification to take place it is difficult to be objective again, to withdraw emotionally. But to be of use to the patient the doctor needs to do just this. He needs to be able to oscillate between the empathic position beside the patient and that of the more detached professional observer.

Work within the group helped the presenting doctor to make further observations about the encounter. The group clarified that the relationship was useful to the patient, although both doctor and patient were unwilling to move into more painful subject matter and work there. It also clarified where some of the emotions appeared to be misplaced. It seemed that this doctor, having identified with the patient, was unable to withdraw into a position of observation without bringing some of the patient's emotions with her. The doctor had been left with profound unease after the consultation, surely she should have – at least – known about the wife's death. The group helped the doctor to locate the strength of that emotion more properly within the patient.

E.B.   You feel you ought to have known more about the wife, and we all say you didn't have to know about the wife. I think we get this terribly wrong if we think, if we know more we are better doctors. You want to know as much as the patient wants you to know, and that's the difficult thing to judge . . .

Dr R.   I think I am convinced that I ignore things about this man that he possibly wants to bring up. I suppose I think it was just odd that I picked up this thing about the black suit. You see what's so awful is that if I had just conducted it in a normal way, he might never have said it . . . .

E.B.   Our aim should be as doctors to relieve human suffering, let's say to get in touch with pain, to find out where the pain is, and so . . . if you can't do anything about the pain well you've just got to tolerate it, like the patient has and act appropriately. What Dr R. feels is that she didn't get in touch with this man's pain . . . . . .but I did think that there was more unwillingness to see Dr R.'s remorse, which I did begin to see as something which came from the patient's treatment of his wife rather than a reality thing by what she had done over the last few years. And, I mean, sooner or later he should be able to tell you how awful he does feel about that last, how long was it that she was in hospital?

Dr R.   Twenty-four hours.

E.B.   The being carried out and the ambulance.

Dr N.   I had a picture of him being at home, not having the courage to go to hospital and then getting a phone call a timeless time later to say that she was dead.

Most of this encounter, quite appropriately, was carried out at the inter-personal level. But this straightforward level of interaction is at times complicated by irrational and unconscious forces which intrude in different ways into the doctor–patient relationship. The leader, particularly if an analyst, will tend to be aware of these patterns. They are usually left undisturbed but on occasion will need discussion if the group work can't move on otherwise.

CONNECTIONS, NARRATIVE AND REVERIE

The second theme that is of importance to the work of the group is personal narrative. The narrative may be jumbled and disordered, and the connec-tions in the threads of the story difficult for the patient or the doctor to follow. Usually in the group the important connections to make relate to the life and feelings of the patient; but at times the group may need to make connections in the doctor's narrative, and occasionally in both at the same time. Our unconsidered thoughts and actions, the things we forget, and the patterns in our dreams and relationships are not simply neurological garbage, but are an important manifestation of the narrative or meaning in our lives, and hence are worth attention and respect.

Some examples of how things that were forgotten, or had slipped from awareness, clearly affected clinical practice may help to illustrate this. The first example looks at connections made for the doctor.

A patient (Sandra Morgan) came to see her doctor. She had made a late marriage at forty-two, and had attended for a missed period, when it became clear that she was not using the contraceptive pill given by another partner some three months previously. She had been to see two gynaecologists who had given her conflicting views on whether she would be able to get pregnant. She came initially asking to see the more hopeful gynaecologist once again, although she was taking the Clomid supplied by the other one. The doctor was puzzled about what she was asking for, especially as she then said, 'Oh! it doesn't matter, perhaps I'm silly to want to see him'.

Before the presentation of this case to the group there was the following exchange:

Dr L.   My case isn't urgent except the only urgency is that part of the thing is I have the greatest difficulty in actually remembering about her and that is one of the surprises.

Dr H.   Is that you or her?

Dr L.   Well I think it's me. Oh! yes I'm sure it's me, but I don't understand why I have the difficulty. I mean when I actually had to ring the surgery to find out her name, although on one level I would know it very well, but on another I couldn't actually remember it . . . . . . but this, there is a different quality about my difficulty because it isn't only her name, it's all sorts of things.

E.B.   It's really well worth noting when one doesn't remember things, they are really important. This girl's name . . .

Dr L.   Her name is Mrs Sandra Morgan and she's forty-three in a fortnight's time.

All.   What precision, what memory!

Eventually, in the discussion, it emerged that this doctor was the first child of a mother of forty-four; the thought of him not being born briefly circulated around the group. The doctor recognised this as helping him to understand why he couldn't remember much about her, or tolerate the thought of her not wanting a baby.

Connections can be easy to make, and nothing is easier than to create a story for the patient which may ease the doctor but which does not generate the narrative tension for doctor and patient to go forward together. One of the functions of the group is to try out different narratives and to be sceptical and questioning about the value of connections made for a patient.

The following part of a transcript comes from the fifth case report of a young woman who had been to her doctor frequently, at first with vaginal discharge and later on with stomach pains and difficulty swallowing. She had told the doctor about a very neglected childhood. She had often run away and even slept in dustbins, and had been raped at the age of eighteen.

Dr R. And then Sharon came in again . . . and what she wanted to talk to me about then was a dream she'd had, which she said had frightened her, which was about how she'd skinned her cat and eaten it, and she was both disgusted at it and confused and I said, 'That must be very unpleasant and frightening for you'. Well, I didn't know where to go from there with her. I was very aware that I didn't want to make any stupid interpretation – well not stupid – jump in and make an interpretation, just to hold on, so that she could tell me about this dream, this sort of happening. And then we turned to talking about her mother, and her quest to find her mother . . . .

Dr H. What do you think it meant?

Dr R. Well I'm sure she feels – well what I think is that she is very worried about how she damages . . . . .

E.B. Damages?

Dr R. Whatever she touches she damages, skins it, eats it, destroys it or whatever.

Dr H. I thought she was the one who was being damaged?

Dr R. She is, it's reciprocal. I mean she is getting damaged so it must be because she is damaging them.

E.B. People who have been damaged are also doing the damage . . . .

Dr H. I think this is phoney. Does it help Ruth to get . . .

Dr L. What's phoney?

Dr H. This so called putting it together and this way, and this is the reciprocal of that . . . .

Dr L. Oh, I see.

Dr H. Now, it could be true, but it doesn't ring a bell with me, but you're the one who is in the driving seat. Does it make you feel better and advance your understanding and help you with patient care?

E.B. What do you mean? You think it's phoney to put together one session with another or one association with another?

Dr H. Unless Ruth can test it by in some way inviting the patient to say more so that she can confirm it I don't see it will remain other than speculation. But that may have done.

E.B.   Speculation isn't necessarily phoney.

Dr R.   I think having some sort of hypothesis about what's going on does help you. Now the problem is it can also be an awful hindrance because you can be barking up the wrong tree and so not listen to what she actually says, and it's quite difficult to be aware of which you're doing.

But what sort of connections might be made for this patient? As doctors we tended to feel out of our depth with this sort of subject matter. We felt bound by the approach to physical causality that our training gives us, and repeatedly experienced difficulties in crossing between the categories of mind and body, often feeling blocked by the idea of speculation, association and connection. It was left to the analyst to make a constructive connection which linked the medical symptom and the dream together, without making an interpretation.

E.B.   This is a particularly difficult one though, isn't it, because she has been complaining about not being able to swallow, and patients can get to a stage where they can't swallow . . . . I mean one could say, 'no wonder you can't swallow if you have that kind of dream', and no more, but there is a connection between her symptom and her dream. But you went on to say about trying to find her mother, which is what she came to tell you about . . . .
. . . . [and a little later]

Dr H.   Well I hope our research will come up with the answer to the question – How long can a doctor carry uncertainty about not knowing what it means? Is what I would term 'spurious certainty' better than remaining puzzled and knowing you know not?

Dr L.   When you say spurious are you categorising what I understood Enid to say as spurious? It seems to me that here is a woman who has had difficulty swallowing, actually talks about swallowing her skinned cat in her dream. It seems to me that it is self-evident that they are both to do with swallowing things and therefore the connection to say, you know, 'If you have ghastly dreams like that no wonder you have difficulty with swallowing'.

Only through repeated follow-ups can the group get a feel for whether connections of this nature help the patient; their value for the doctor in making the patient's story more coherent is seen more easily.

The third example shows how the doctor and patient's narrative can sometimes get emotionally entangled; sorting out the connections for one can bring relief for both. Jill Norman, a twenty-three-year-old epileptic girl was seen by her doctor when she was about twenty weeks' pregnant. She had concealed it and expressed concern that the baby would be taken away. She attended a day centre, and during the doctor's absence the staff arranged for a termination.

A few months later she began to attend her general practitioner more frequently with complaints of bleeding, abdominal pains and nausea. After six months of such consultations, the doctor realised that she had been unable to ask her how she felt about the termination. On asking, the patient graphically described her loss, and got some relief from her symptoms.

The doctor was amazed at her incomprehensible delay at making the obvious link and talking about her patient's feelings. During the discussion in the group it became known that the doctor had had a miscarriage at about the same time the patient had had a termination. For some months the emotions in the doctor had prevented her making connections for the patient which were later to help her with her symptoms. The key point is that the doctor remained unaware of why she was doing this until late on in the group discussion.

PACE AND DIRECTION

The third important theme shared with psychoanalysis is self-exploration. That is, giving the patient time and encouragement in the context of a professional relationship to reflect on what things mean for them, at a depth and pace of their own choosing. This is an approach that is widely applied within most counselling or psychotherapeutic settings, but needs a conscious effort to incorporate within the setting of general practice. Within the short encounters of a surgery session it is often extremely difficult to clear away the emotions belonging to the previous case or to a distracting phone call and be available for the next patient. But in spite of this, as the following example shows, the doctor's response to the patient can be finely tuned and quite specific in its intention. Recall the case of Mrs Susan Towle, first mentioned in Chapter 1, which can be summarized as follows:

Dr L. saw fifty-eight-year-old Susan, whom he had known for thirty years as a jokey bus conductress. When her husband dropped dead from a heart attack, she came to see him, greatly distressed at having seen his body after a mutilating post-mortem examination. Dr L. was profoundly affected by her grief, realising that he had misdiagnosed the depth of her emotional life for a very long time.

She came back after two weeks, at first being something of her jokey self, saying she had an attack of her bronchiectasis. The doctor asked why she had not called and she said, 'Oh, well you're busy'. The doctor then said how distressed he had been to see how she was last time, 'I've known you thirty years and felt I've never known you at all'. She then cried, and said how she wanted to be looked after just now.

The doctor saw her several more times, attempting to help by providing sick certificates and letting her decide the pace of contacts.

At a much later group meeting there was a discussion of this presentation, with the question of why this case was so surprising. We all see people and suddenly become aware of different aspects of them. We catch glimpses of this and that about them, not understanding a person in depth but gradually catching up with a reasonably consistent picture of them.

Dr B. But with Susan she was changing, with a very dramatic experience in her life. Possibly she looked in the coffin and thought suddenly – My God, I never knew my husband or he never knew me – and that was Leonard's surprise. He was devastated, I feel, by the experience of not knowing her, and maybe that was in part also something to do with what Susan herself was experiencing.

E.B. Susan was coming across something strange in herself picked up by L . . . .

Dr L. . . . . and it was this sudden change that she threw at me, and I caught it.

Dr L. felt that his relationship with the patient had remained altered, more relaxed and honest, a contrast with his feelings after the first presented consultation. Had the group played any part in this?

Dr L. I think it had something to do, I do. I remember part of the group discussion, I remember the spirit of the group discussion; and certainly I think it was helpful because I came locked in my own pain, which was Susan's pain, and certainly I think the group discussion allowed me to see ways forward.

The doctor didn't explain to Susan what was going on. Indeed, he couldn't, because he couldn't know from the fragments he was given. But the doctor did make observations – to himself, and to the group – about his own altered feelings, and made use of those observations quite intentionally during the next consultation. This enabled Susan to say how she wanted to be looked after. The doctor didn't try explaining this either, although it might have been tempting to try. Instead, he made a number of moves that helped her to have the experience of being looked after, and in consecutive consultations she was able to show the doctor that she was looking at bits of life that had been affected by her husband's death.

Within the group, similar work was proceeding. The doctor brought his distress about the case to the group, and he was gradually brought to see that the depressed mood belonged more properly in Susan than in himself. But the change in the patient had affected the doctor such that there was a change in him too. The context of their relationship had been permanently altered. Moments of change for both patients and doctors may be times when productive new practices or attitudes can be incorporated; work in Balint groups fosters moments such as these, and so encourages change.

TIMESCALE, SETTING AND VOCABULARY

There are two further themes which are important within both the psycho-analytic tradition and general practice. These are timescale and the setting or context. In both disciplines the timescale is a long one. Changes within individuals in general practice can often be seen only over a period of years; indeed, as the last case illustrates, it may be years into a relationship before the occasion arises for a significant revelation, or for the doctor and patient to be jolted out of their usual mode of working. The setting of general practice is clearly very different from that of analytic or psychotherapeutic practice. As doctors of first contact we are in a position to observe how our patients use us, to pay attention to the beginnings and endings of contacts and to repeated consultations. General practitioners are often involved in different types of task at the same time; an acute illness may intervene and change the pace of a long-running contact, or an encounter with another family member may illuminate a patient's problems. As general practi-tioners we need to observe the value of the setting in which we work, and to pay attention to developing its particular virtues. The advantages of being a generalist are especially important, allowing the focus of attention in the consultation to remain within a strictly medical vocabulary if that is where the patient is most comfortable; but using that familiar language to reach into areas that might otherwise be too distressing for either doctor or patient to discuss more clearly. Examples of this were quite frequently seen within the work of the group, as the following case illustrates.

Ann Shipman, a quiet and unobtrusive girl of fifteen, had been with the practice all her life, hardly ever attending. When she came to see her doctor on this occasion she said the problem was that she had a lot of upper stomach pains and it had been really bad over the weekend. She said that her mum and dad were separated and she lived with her dad who had a duodenal ulcer. She also said that her dad thought it might be due to stresses. She was not forthcoming about the stresses, only saying that she was not a worrier. The doctor gave her some symptomatic treatment and was left wondering. When she came back it was no better. She was still unforthcoming, but sat looking at the doctor wanting something done. Reluctantly the doctor ordered a barium meal, saying she expected it to be normal, as indeed it was. After this they returned again, as in each consultation, to things at home. She said that she sees her mum quite often, and then she said with enormous feeling, 'I can't stand the way they hate each other'. She expressed it all in that statement and it became transparently clear where the problem was as she described how she felt torn apart by loving them both.

Afterwards in the group there was a lot of discussion about the doctor's anxiety about arranging the barium meal. There was talk about the feeling of pressure to do something, of the use of a test to 'look inside' a withholding patient, and the professional correctness of such a decision:

Dr H.   It may be that until the barium meal had been done it's not that the patient didn't speak about it but that you didn't hear.

E.B.   Indeed. I'm not at all convinced that this couldn't have been done without the barium meal, but I just can't see in my innocence that it is such a terrible price to pay.

However, it was the psychoanalyst within the group who helped to affirm the value of the medical vocabulary of general practice, and to help the doctor to use it:

E.B.   It was the way she said 'I cannot stand . . . hatred'. Of course I could have said she has to talk about her own hatred and her hatred of herself and so on; but hatred has been raised as the ulcer, hasn't it?

In this case the doctor moved at the patient's pace from the somatic to the psychic content of her distress, and this was clearly seen in the change in the patient's vocabulary. The doctor and the group expressed their difficulties in making this transition by focusing on 'professional' questions, such as the proper uses of resources. The underlying concern was about responding to patients' psychological distress presented in somatic forms. It would seem that the general practitioner was indeed 'ideally placed' to work with this patient in her distress – a counsellor would have been at a great disadvantage. It was truly whole-person medicine.

This way of working, using some of the insights gained from a psychoanalytic approach, and many of the advantages of the general practice setting, has helped doctors to become aware of areas of their work which they might otherwise ignore. The group working together can help the doctors to be more observant of themselves, particularly of their emotional reactions, and hence to become more observant of their patients.

Part II

Observations and surprises

4 The work of a psychoanalyst in Balint groups

> Perhaps the most important factor is the behaviour of the leader of the group . . . By allowing everybody to be themselves, to have their say in their own way and in their own time, by watching for proper cues – that is, speaking only when something is *really* expected from him and making his point in a form which, instead of prescribing *the* right way, opens up possibilities for the doctors to discover themselves *some* right way . . .
>
> (Balint 1957:306)

In this chapter we will consider the work of a psychoanalyst within the group. We have wondered whether the psychoanalyst's task as leader might generate difficulties for him as a thinker and a worker. But the presence of a psychoanalyst – with that particular way of looking at people and groups of people, with an awareness of unconscious processes, and a familiarity with paradoxes and contradictions – might widen the perspective and ways of thinking in a group, especially a group which has been educated to see its patients in one way: mostly in terms of illnesses; to answer the questions, 'what is wrong and how can I put it right?'

We realised from the start that an analyst who has not been subjected to the thinking, feeling, despair and pleasure of general practitioners was not equipped to lead a Balint group. Likewise, a general practitioner who wants to lead a Balint seminar needs to have been subjected to the thinking of an analyst who has worked with general practitioners for some years. The education is mutual; neither is capable of doing the other's job. Analyst-leaders are needed who have been trained by general practitioners and general practitioner-leaders need training by analysts.

However, before deciding on the use of a psychoanalyst in a Balint group, we need to describe briefly again what task the group is assembled to carry out. One could say that the task is to help general practitioners in their professional life: to make them feel more at ease with their patients and with themselves as doctors so that they can help their patients more constructively with less stress.

This task cannot be done by psychoanalysts who wish to teach their theories, but rather by those who are interested in using themselves more like a clinician in a professional setting. They need to be as alert as they are with their patients, and not jump to conclusions too quickly. They need to be ready to let the group do the work, helping mainly by telling the group what it has said rather than by interpreting underlying meanings. The doctor must know that he has reached this understanding himself and that it arises out of what he says, rather than by what has been put into him like a foreign body. The psychoanalyst is there as a facilitator – an opener of doors – not as an instructor. Both psychoanalyst and general practitioners have to pay attention and listen to what happens in the surgery, because it is only from the memory of events in the surgery that both can learn and rethink and change perspectives and build up a picture that enlightens. Neither can learn by being told what to do.

It has been pointed out in this book that we believe in the value of subjective ideas about reality. We do not rule out such ideas simply because they are subjective but take them into account and see whether we can learn from them. It is necessary to have a personal view to make sense of the world. This idea is accepted in Balint seminars but perhaps not in other general practitioner groups with different aims. Our aim, we repeat, is to widen perspectives in a useful way: to help doctors see more without ignoring what they already know. Their focus of attention might change, but they do not cease to give attention to the things which they gave attention to before.

So then, in what ways does a psychoanalyst contribute to the work in the group? Analysts are trained, or train themselves, to wait before commenting, and they do not jump to conclusions. Everybody will say, 'But they have plenty of time; they work for years with patients.' However, general practitioners can waste part of their 'six minutes' if they feel harassed or that some simple explanation of some puzzling complaint should be found. This may make them want to intervene at an early stage, in which case they may in fact lose time as they may fail to hear what is important, which indeed may be something quite simple, something which is told in such a way that the doctor could easily fail to hear it. Or the patient may indeed have failed to tell the doctor something which he has not noticed was omitted from the story. We have had examples of that in this book (in the case of Mr Jennings).

The analyst, because of his training and theories, is bound to see things about relationships or the private life of the patient, or the absence of information or the excess of it, more quickly than the general practitioner;

analogously, the analyst knows that the general practitioner will see much more quickly than he does what is physically wrong with the patient and how to manage it.

The fact, however, that the analyst does see something useful does not mean that he wants to talk about it and possibly shift the emphasis in a way which might leave out the general practitioner's observations. He has to wait until he thinks that it is appropriate or might lead to some understanding which is not out of keeping with other observations but may lead the group to work with a different aspect of the patient.

This is illustrated in the discussion about Sandra Morgan (first discussed in Chapter 3). The first thing her doctor said was that he had difficulty in remembering her name and other things about her. At this point, before he went on to explain that she had married late, aged forty-two, and came with a mixed message about wanting and not wanting to be pregnant, the leader interrupted like this:

E.B.   It's really well worth noting when one doesn't remember things, they are really important.

Much later in the discussion, when the group was trying to understand why this doctor was struggling so much, the leader changed the direction of the discussion from a focus on what led him to forget the patient, like this:

E.B   . . . the fact that you really have not told us anything about this girl at all apart from her sterility or pre-menopausal state is very strange. It isn't that you forgot her name, I think one forgets names for a variety of reasons – unless she reminds you of somebody else – but you *don't know* her.

Dr L.   I've only seen her three times.

Until then the group had colluded with the idea that the doctor had just forgotten things about this woman rather than never having known them or found it difficult to know her.

Analysts are trained to stay with an idea and to be able to tolerate uncertainty. We think it is likely that analysts or people who have worked with analysts and are therefore in touch with their pace of work and their ability to hold on to information (which many people would prefer to verbalise quickly) can change the variety of ways in which a patient can be treated. In a later chapter we cite the example of how various people sitting in a room might look at an apple suspended from the ceiling. They would see different sides of the apple and together they would see the whole. Of course, we have not forgotten that doctors in their work with patients in the organic field are quite used to holding on to observations and taking a look from different angles; and that they are trained to think about when to discuss a particular symptom or illness with a patient and when to wait. They are not in a hurry to tell patients about their findings. But they might be unfamiliar with the strain of holding on to information or hypotheses or inferences about the patient's attitude to himself and to other people which might be making it difficult to function. Many things are too hard to bear.

Analysts can also contribute to the group by demonstrating an approach which stands aside from, or transcends, any particular theory. At the beginning of their career many analysts may pay too much attention to a particular theory because of their lack of understanding. Observations are too difficult to make where there is no theory to back them up. But theory has to be kept in abeyance when working with patients. Two examples will show the effect of this, both in work with the patient and in work within the group.

Ann, a girl of fifteen, last discussed in Chapter 3, had been a patient of the practice all her life. She had been consulting more frequently in the last four years, complaining of stomach pains and dysmenorrhoea. She had been prescribed an oral contraceptive preparation for the latter. She presented as a very quiet, quite attractive girl with long blonde hair, though she always slipped into the consulting room unobtrusively. At a recent consultation she complained of stomach pain. It seemed unrelated to eating – simple measures such as milk and indigestion tablets had not relieved it. She volunteered that her father had a history of duodenal ulcer and so had her brother and uncle. She wondered if she was developing an ulcer like her father, though he, himself, had thought it was her 'nerves'. Physical examination revealed no signs, and the question of her nerves was discussed, but revealed nothing. A barium meal was arranged, and at follow-up she was told the barium meal was normal. It then emerged that her parents were divorcing after having been separated for four years. She had lived with her father during this time. She said, 'I can't stand the way they hate each other'. It was clear that she was torn apart inside because she loved them both and could not bear them running each other down when she was with one of them; and she seemed able to accept that her bottled up emotions might well be the cause of her symptoms. It was noteworthy that her increased attendance had occurred since her parents separated.

She might have liked very much to be told that her pains were because of her attachment to her father, but such theoretical interpretation would not have helped her long term, though it might have diverted her attention from her pain for a while. But it would not have made her stronger or less anxious. Her future would not have seemed less hopeless. It was essential that she, herself, made the connection between her physical pain and her distress over her parents splitting up.

The second example shows a similar sort of principle at work, but this time between the members of the group. We have met the patient concerned in Chapter 3.

Sharon, a young woman of twenty-five, had been introduced to her doctor by her probation officer, as she was on probation for a minor offence. She had had a deprived childhood, and was half West Indian. She complained of difficulty in eating and swallowing, and occasionally vomiting. There did not seem to be anything seriously wrong, but the doctor was phoned by the probation officer to report that Sharon continued to be worried about her stomach. When she returned to the doctor she wanted to tell her about a dream she had had, which had frightened her. She dreamed that she had skinned her cat and eaten it, and she was both disgusted at it and confused. The doctor said that it must have been very unpleasant and frightening for her, but felt unable to go much further, aware that she didn't want to make an interpretation of the dream, because of feelings of insecurity about her competence to make such interpretations. An extract from the transcript shows how the discussion proceeded.

E.B.   This is a particularly difficult one . . . . she has been complaining about not being able to swallow and patients can get to a stage where they can't swallow. In the dream there is something pretty horrid she's swallowed . . . So by leaving the . . . hidden meaning of the dream, which I don't know about, to look at the manifest,[1] the actual dream . . . is the way forward. Unless you say something about it you are not dealing with her symptom, which is she can't swallow. I think this is a difficult one from that point of view.

Dr R.   Yes.

E.B.   I mean one could say, 'No wonder you can't swallow if you have that kind of dream', and no more: but there is a connection between her symptoms and the dream, which there isn't always.

Dr R.   Mm.

Dr L.   Enid says that remark so that it seems so self-evident . . . . I mean it's so right but I'm not sure I would have perceived . . . . . .

E.B.   The connection between dream and symptom? For a start you'd be thinking, 'God I can't stand dreams'.

Dr R.
and   } That's right.
Dr R.

Dr R.   The theory had obstructed me and prevented me from being spontaneous.

E.B.   Feeling that you don't know the theory, you sit and listen and just sympathise.

Dr L.   Absolutely . . . .

E.B.   This is true all the time.

Dr G.   But what you said, Enid, is so beautifully simple. It only makes the connection as far as it needs to be made. It's not like saying, 'There are two ideas of bad things inside you', or something sophisticated like that.

Dr R.   It's coming out of the other side of all that theory and that's the trouble – we're sort of splashing around in the shallows.

E.B.   I think it is important because we are studying what we can't hear and this is a really good example . . . . .

This illustrates how the analyst, although familiar with the theory of dream interpretation, can show that a complicated theory is not needed to make connections using dreams which may be useful for the patient.

Analysts can hold on to contradictory and paradoxical ideas without discarding one or the other. Contradictory ideas need to flourish and to be maintained within the framework of ideas of the group. The analyst needs to choose the right moment to introduce them to the group and be able to follow the response.

Two examples of how an analyst can help to hold contradictory ideas within the group also come from transcripts of the case of Sharon. She had initially presented to her doctor with symptoms of vaginal discharge. She kept getting trichomonal infection although it appeared to have been treated appropriately both by her general practitioner and a clinic for sexually transmitted diseases she attended. She repeatedly said she did not have a current boyfriend.

Dr L.   But if she does come back to you, she probably will, with the vaginal discharge, what then? . . .

Dr R.   You see I think the conflicting messages that are coming across to me from her is that I have this fantasy that she must be sexually active, and yet all the talk all the time is about how can she possibly have intercourse because of the awful thing she's going to give them, so there's a conflicting message and I don't quite know where I am with it. It's very difficult to know where to pick it up, or does she really not want to talk about it.

Dr I.   Well, that's what she says, but does she perhaps mean how can she enjoy it? . . .

E.B.   How can she? I mean with her – like someone says, 'How can I possibly have a hundred cigarettes a day?' I mean how can one? But one does. If one could only get her to assume if she does, then one could get her to talk about how it is and where it is. How to get over this awful thing, because once a patient says 'No, I never do masturbate', or I never do whatever it is, you're stuck, you can't do anything, and you, if possible, want to put them in a position of not having to lie to you. She does lie, she always has, we're assuming that. I don't know, how to get her so that she can go back – I mean how Ruth can assume that she does have intercourse or she is promiscuous or whatever . . . . .

The second example comes much later in the case. The patient's symptoms had moved from her vagina to her stomach; when she had presented the doctor with dreams about skinning and eating her cat, and there had been an extensive search to find her mother. Then everything seemed to go quiet, the doctor felt she was marking time, and then the patient came again after a gap of several months with no real change. There was a feeling in the group that work should be pressing ahead, and there was a lot of interrogation of the doctor seeking for new material.

E.B.   I mean the point surely for us is whether Ruth wants to, should or wants to let this girl talk about – I don't know what . . . . .

Dr H.   Well, we don't have transcripts of consultations and we don't know what this girl says but only what Ruth heard.

E.B.   Well, we know how Ruth feels, which is all we're interested in.

Dr H.   Well, now you're speculating why didn't the girl come for six months?

E.B.   Yes, well we don't know.

Dr H.   Well, there's a possible theory which is the girl was trying to say something and it was not heard.

Dr L.   The other thing of course is the opposite, is in fact she got what she wanted from Ruth which lasted six months.

Dr H.   I don't know. How do you react when patients don't come back to us? Is it a cure? . . .

Dr R.   Henry you were saying that she was telling me things but I wasn't hearing them and I'm not quite sure what you think I wasn't hearing apart from maybe the sexual . . . .

Dr H.   Still, I don't know if Ruth's heard it but she's come back after six months with a variety of tickets of entry, none of which seem particularly genuine, and that does raise the speculation is this her second time round trying? I don't know . . . .

E.B.   I think one of the difficulties about this, one of the difficulties is that in one part of our minds we're thinking that if this case is brought to a group we should cure the patient. Well this patient is incurable isn't she in one way? We're not going to give her what she didn't have for the first twenty-five years of her life, and all you or we can do is make it a bit easier for her. I can't see how we would expect to change her, but we could make it a bit easier and I think you did for a time, so perhaps you can again. I don't know whether I was picking up something wrong but I think we were thinking that we should see to it that she settles down with a nice chap and lives happily ever after. There's not the remotest chance of this is there? She might in five or ten years be better, but Ruth can help her on her way.

Dr R.   Yes, and I think that's quite helpful because I think I am, and I think other people here are trying to make me find, listen, whatever it is, the cause somehow of what's turned her funny. And maybe there isn't any more in what she's telling me than what is there.

By drawing out and expressing these contradictory ideas the analyst reminded the group that a patient's story is rarely sequential. Instead, there are conflicting and often paradoxical aims and desires which can be a source of confusion and frustration for the doctor.

Within the work of the group a similar effect can be noted. The group longs for an explicable story, with initial causes and a suitable outcome, and may seek supporting details from the material brought by the presenting doctor. The analyst needs to remind the group of the painful and contradictory elements of the story so that the group can observe the doctor and patient in a more realistic way.

A final example from the same case shows the analyst-leader working in the group to help with ideas about timing and the appropriate time to put words to feelings. During an earlier consultation the patient, Sharon (see Chapter 3), had described how her stepmother had been cruel and she frequently used to run away.

Dr R   ... and the thing that really sticks with me is that she said, 'I used to run away and I'd sleep anywhere, I'd sleep in the dustbin', a terribly tragic sort of moment really. And eventually she ran away and put herself in care .... It was quite an intimate consultation, I certainly felt very moved by the end of it, and the thing about this dustbin really stuck with me. I felt that really showed how she felt about herself, that she was rubbish.

E.B.   But you didn't say?

Dr R.   I did to some extent, I said, 'You must have felt awful and unwanted'.

E.B.   You didn't say rubbish? . . . . .

Dr R.   You see she has told me some of this before and I think the change in me is that I can now remember it clearly and therefore it's obviously – it means more to me . . . . .

E.B.   If people can say the same thing over and over again to you then it means absolutely nothing and it isn't that you can't hear but because it isn't appropriate to you . . . . .

Dr H. I must say I don't share the general opinion that you failed in your professionalism by not mentioning the famous phrase 'you must have felt like rubbish'. . . . . . But it seemed to me you transcended this by being rooted to the spot and just listening . . . . .

E.B. I think there is an awful lot to talk about because the thing is that I don't think it would be routine to say you felt like rubbish, depends on how you said it but is there any value and if so, of putting – of naming something on their level, and I think there is actually, but it's the timing of it that's important. I think putting a name, putting a word to something for the first time is terribly important. This girl had never used that word about herself, she had all these symptoms but I think there's a lot to be said for not having done it then, but I think we could talk about when is it valuable to use a word.

Dr H. I'm getting increasingly doubtful about the value of words. I know we were brought up to say this and that and to make the correct interpretations.

E.B. But that's not using the word to the patient. I mean to use the right word for the patient is not making interpretations is it? It's just finding a word. It's not saying you did something because of something, it's letting something be said. It's quite different you know in my view.

Dr H. Did Ruth feel confident that it was rubbish the girl was expressing or just awfulness? . . . .

Dr R. Yes of course it was and I think, well I did, I stepped back from . . . . .

E.B. There's such a lot here about what comes from oneself and what's put into oneself from the patient and to sort this out on any occasion it's very, very difficult. I think this sort of discussion opens it up and we can have a look.

The importance of finding the right language was discussed several times. The accuracy with which the doctor and the patient can name the feelings and events in the consultation will reflect not only the quality of observations, but also whether the doctor and the patient have got close enough to allow the emergence of such thoughts and feelings.

This description of the use of the analyst in the group is of course only partial. The focus has been on what the general practitioners themselves thought was of particular value. The way we used language, and questions of timing and holding on to our observations were issues raised directly by the case material; whilst questions about theory, as a help or hindrance and the ability to hold on to paradoxical ideas, came largely out of the group work.

When an analyst is also the leader further questions arise. Can the analyst's intervention – his ability to show the doctor what he can stand, or to show him how he might be limiting his patients by the way that he works – be of use? Can this perhaps be of help or is the doctor best left on his own to find his strengths and weaknesses and to live with them?

Observers, as we have often said, affect and change what they observe. We know from many sources that patients learn how doctors like them to behave and what sort of illnesses they really like them to have. Doctors also have their own interests and strengths and they encourage their patients along certain lines without knowing it. This is inevitable. Both patient and doctor are constantly influenced by each other and by what they can hear or by what they can bear to hear. Should the aim of the analyst-leader be to help the doctors live with their own limitations and not get too depressed or elated by their successes or failures? This demonstrates some of the difficulties the analyst as leader faces in deciding when to intervene to help doctors gain an insight into the nature of their own professional work, which is not primarily by giving insight into the psychological causes of a patient's illness or the techniques needed to manage them. It is essential for the leader not to imply that the doctor should be able to tune into every patient. It is also important that the analyst is able to experience and show how little he can understand at any given moment, and be willing to be wrong without embarrassment even in his own field. After all, he also has blind spots and defences and things he cannot bear.

The most important thing the leader of a Balint group must do is to be prepared to watch his own and the doctors' observations and ways of reacting to errors and to misconceptions, and to work with them in order to understand the patient and his illness. We came to the conclusion quite early in our work that the doctor had to be ready to be surprised. Unless he can be surprised at his own reactions as well as those of his patients then he cannot learn, but may instead try to rid his work of the subjective which would mean that he would be left having to think 'rationally' all the time.

It is necessary for the analyst sometimes to come in with a comment about the observer-error or the group's desire to chase some quite unprofitable hare in order to avoid looking at what is quite simply in the foreground. When he does this he must know what he is doing and wait for various responses from the group. So the analyst-leader has to be in touch with not only subjective responses between the patient and the doctor, but also his own response and then the group's reaction to that.

Finally, it is important to stress the mutuality of the experience between the doctors in the group and the analyst-leader. The general practitioners' ideas and observations have as much importance as the leader's. Neither has priority; they work as equals. The leader needs a group; a group needs a leader. And in our view a psychoanalyst, who is close to the physicians with whom he works (not personally but professionally), is a help rather than a hindrance. Balint groups started with and have not given up the idea that psychoanalysts do contribute to work done in such a group and to the skills which may develop out of it. We could even say that partnership between members of the two disciplines has been the essence of our method of work.

NOTE

1 Used here to mean the remembered not the latent content of the dream.

5 Taking the observer-error seriously

In the last resort, it is a matter of how one makes headway in biology. I think that the feeling of wonder which physicists had thirty years ago has taken a new turn. Life will always be a wonder, but what changes is the balance between the feeling of wonder and the courage to understand.

(Bohr 1963:29)

The next two chapters take a new route through the Balints' ideas taking into account general scientific concepts. The traditional approach of medical education can be narrow and preoccupied with certainty and the exclusive pursuit of 'objectivity'. Medicine can isolate itself by this line of enquiry, which the behavioural sciences consider counterproductive and the basic sciences increasingly regard as producing diminishing returns. Relinquishing these ideas and taking a more pragmatic approach led the group to a new starting place and a course that was only charted after the research seminars had finished, but which began during the group discussions. It sprang from this remark:

Perhaps the most important item of thought which the Balints brought to general practice was – *to take the observer-error seriously in order to incorporate it into an understanding of the patient and his illness.*

There are two notions at the centre of this statement: the 'observer-error' and 'taking it seriously'. They offer an opportunity to examine the importance of the personal bias that every doctor brings to every observation or decision he makes – the observer-error – and also to study the incorporation of this in the Balint working method – that is, the taking it seriously. Both are rooted in the belief that observation is at the heart of good practice and that we all bring a personal view to what we observe, which needs attention. This personal dimension should be valued and not dismissed as misleading or unscientific. On the contrary, the doctor's subjective view may be very valuable to the patient, provided it is used appropriately. Balint groups help doctors to learn about and understand the way they respond so that they can then use it to the patient's advantage. The purpose of this chapter is to look in detail at that method to provide a context to describe and examine the small but important shifts in our group's way of working.

It should be made clear that the emphasis in this chapter will be on the method used by the group and not on the individual techniques used by the doctors with their patients. Since the aim of working together in a group like this is to help doctors modify their methods so that they are more helpful to their patients, the reader will want to see this demonstrated. This sequence of events can be difficult to show. The modification of a doctor's technique may take time or occasionally be shown by a single exchange with a patient, but either way there may be a delay before it can be shown to be of use to the patient. In this chapter we want to look at the first link in the chain – how the group's observations help the doctor. We will try, where we can, to link the two and show how helping the doctor helped the patient.

Balint seminars are guided by a simple and elegant concept. This is to examine the relationship between the doctor and the patient, to look at the feelings generated in the doctor as possibly being part of the patient's world, and then use this to help the patient. If these feelings do not seem to belong to the patient but to the doctor, it helps to know that too. To be a participant in a relationship and also its observer is fraught with difficulties and potential bias. The aim is to study this carefully. As a consequence doctors can take the feelings that arise from their work seriously and pay attention to much that would otherwise be disregarded. The Balints were the first to introduce the idea of the participant observer into the arena of clinical medicine.

The theory may be simple but its execution is not. Looking at feelings is not plain sailing. The Balints developed a framework within which to pursue these ideas, which they called a 'research-cum-training' seminar. The traditionally trained medical scientist might find it paradoxical to combine training, which implies change and development, with research, which suggests some sort of stability in the observer. However, what the Balints meant by this epithet was quite straightforward. It was to find out what general practice was like and whether they could help throw light on the subject and explore new techniques and methods of working (Balint 1984:2). They did not come to teach or tell general practitioners what to do, but genuinely to explore the discipline. The aim of the training is not as many would suppose to define the psychological cause of the patient's distress but to be clear about the observations made by the doctor. The training is to be precise about what is observed. If the doctor is uncertain about what has been observed, or if there are inconsistencies in the observations, then it is worth being quite clear about this. The aim of the research is to see if this is of any professional use to general practitioners.

Nowadays, many general practitioners have had some experience of small groups in which an atmosphere of exploration prevails. However, the freedom generated in a Balint group is for a well-defined purpose, so that the doctors can look and listen to what is going on inside as well as outside themselves. This is one of the features that distinguishes a Balint seminar from other small groups. If the boundaries of a group are clearly defined, not too constricting and, most importantly, stable, then a freedom arises in which professional feelings can be examined. What is aimed for is an openness and honesty and in particular an ability to hold back and not rush in too quickly to find explanations. Furthermore, fresh observations are encouraged in order to break out of the professional tendency which leads us to observe only what we already understand.

The seminar provides a stable setting to explore the vocabulary of the doctor's feelings within the framework of his relationship with his patient. Usually about eight to ten general practitioners meet with a psychoanalyst leader and sometimes a general practitioner co-leader, who has experience of Balint seminars; all anticipate making at least a two-year commitment to meet for about an hour and a half every week of academic term time. The doctors are asked to talk about any patient with whom they are having difficulties or who interests them particularly, preferably not about patients with obvious neurotic or psychotic illness, but ordinary patients, whom they have seen in their practices. They are not asked to present their patients from their notes but from memory. This may at first sight seem odd, but it allows the doctors to speak more freely, contradict themselves, forget and then remember things. It enables the doctors to emphasise those things they feel are important rather than just those which they record in an orderly way. Forgetting and remembering in this way is unlikely to arise in the course of a more conventional case discussion, and if it does it often gives rise to embarrassment, which prevents it being used easily. However, in a Balint group these sorts of happenings are valued because they can indicate important feelings the doctors have about their patients, which they may keep hidden even from themselves. These emerge in a natural way if the group is relaxed and free enough. Each member will notice different points and in the ensuing discussion will share their observations and ideas, paying particular attention to aspects that were overlooked both by the doctor with the patient and by the group in their discussion. Contradictions are examined. Observations are separated from inferences and the doctor is encouraged to tell the group as much as he knows about the patient, including what may seem quite trivial thoughts which arise during the course of the seminar.

Paying this sort of attention to patients can be novel for doctors. As medical students we are taught that if we can identify the cause of an illness we are more likely to be able to help the patient. By the time doctors become general practitioners they realise that cause is not the only aspect to understanding illness. Those unable to accept this can find it difficult to tolerate the confusion and uncertainty in general practice, where causes are rarely precisely identified. This uncertainty about cause does not prevent general practitioners from looking after their patients. What stops doctors caring appropriately is when they fail to observe their patients closely. All clinicians know this when managing physical illness, for example, in distinguishing between left ventricular failure and asthma. If after examining the patient the doctor is unable to decide between these two, a chest X-ray, which extends the clinical description, is likely to be helpful. This principle is central to the Balint method and aims to shift the focus of doctors from one of searching for causes to one of paying more attention to observation.

An example of this is given by Dr N. when he first presented his patient Aurora, a thirty-two-year-old mineralogist. He had known her well for two years since she had had her second child. At that time she had booked her confinement in the local hospital and importantly, at her request, this was to be under Dr N.'s care in the general practitioner unit. She had had a post-partum haemorrhage after the birth of her first child and, furthermore, her own mother had died in her second confinement, four hours after Aurora was born. In the event Aurora's second child was born precipitately at home. An ambulance, which had been called, was left waiting 'just in case'. The labour, although rapid, had been followed by a good delivery and accompanied by a delightful family scene with father present and the first child soon invited in to see that all was well. In the light of this, after an hour, the ambulance was sent away. Soon after this Aurora began to bleed and was rushed to hospital by an emergency ambulance where she received four pints of blood and sutures to her torn cervix. All seemed well but on the fifth day she started to bleed again, was re-admitted and needed further surgical intervention for retained placental material. In the next few months Aurora deteriorated, with marked weight loss and episodes of severe abdominal pain. No effort was spared in investigation; however, all the blood tests, X-rays, IVP, scans, etc, proved normal.

It was almost twelve months before the doctor made any reference to Aurora about her mother's death, and even then only in passing. Despite being underweight (41 kg and 5 ft 6 inches) and in poor health, Aurora carried on a successful career as a mineralogist at London University, giving learned papers at home and abroad.

A week before Dr N. presented Aurora to the group she had approached him for help to secure twelve months' sabbatical leave to 'enjoy the children'. The university would not oblige and told her to take sick leave. She didn't like that. Instead, she was thinking of applying for a post in the civil service. She wanted, in her own words, 'to be doing something useful instead of just enjoying myself'. Dr N. assured her he would provide whatever certification was needed, and while on the point of leaving the room in search for forms for further investigations he heard her say, 'I'm sure there is a lot of psychosomatic stuff down there'. He was unable to stop and stay in the room. Returning, he managed to say, 'Like what?' But this fell flat.

That evening Aurora phoned Dr N. at home to confirm that he would provide medical reports for her to take extended sick leave. However, the next morning he found a note from her saying, 'Don't bother to write; I am going to become a civil servant.'

There were several surprises in the group discussion that followed.

Dr L.   I wondered, really, because I thought it unusual for you to have gone and got that bloody form instead of actually staying. What/
Dr J.   It was more painful for Nick to just sit down there and then and take it up.
E.B.   He wanted to get away.
Dr L.   I think he suddenly had a vision of whether he could stand the pain that was going to come out.
Dr N.   Well she bloody nearly died that's the point.
Dr L.   Absolutely.

There was no doubt in the group's mind that the doctor had to get out of the consulting room, although the doctor himself found this difficult to accept at first. The doctor had previously seen the patient as the one unable to discuss things. The group's view redressed that and allowed him to see that he was, at least, as responsible for avoiding things as the patient. It opened the way for him to make use of the second surprise: how little he could recall about the facts the group asked for in their discussion.

E.B.   What sex are the children?
Dr N.   I've forgotten the sex of the second child.
Dr B.   Of the first child?
Dr N.   Of the second child.
Dr B.   Of this one?
Dr N.   The first child was a boy.
Dr I.   You mean this one you delivered. [All laughing]

What an odd thing that he should not know the sex of the child he had delivered! Several felt that it was a reflection of the mother's own distance from her child. Certainly, it might be something to do with mothering and accepting or rejecting that role. An explanation was offered which the group agreed with and seemed to make sense to the doctor:

E.B.   . . . in spite of your closeness and obvious liking for her, you are terrified of being this woman's mother.

Dr N.   Hadn't thought of it like that; because of associations I suppose, yes.

E.B.   Perhaps she – well I don't know what she is doing to make you, she's doing something, she's saying, 'I'll do this alone', isn't she? 'You can't stop me', and you're agreeing in a way? [Dr N.: Yes.] I mean do other people think this is what is going on?

Dr B.   I certainly think the terrifying responsibility of being her mother is central, that is really clear.

Dr N.   Mm, the terrifying responsibility.

Dr R.   But I also think that Nick has been her mother in lots of ways and I think he's done/

E.B.   But not enough.

Dr N.   But the terrifying responsibility of being a doctor as well.

E.B.   Yes, absolutely.

These surprises and connections were useful to the doctor. It was demonstrated quite clearly that the patient rendered Dr N. temporarily ineffective as a doctor. Not only did he forget facts about the patient but he also found it difficult to see connections about her, her illness and himself, until quite near the end of the discussion:

Dr L.   But I think Nick has had surprises in the group work as well as everybody else?

Dr N.   Very much so. In fact I think it's helped me get a distance from it which I haven't had for a long time.

Dr L.   And I think it was that note. The interesting thing is that note, which annoyed him so much. {Meaning the one saying 'don't bother to write the letter; I've decided to become a civil servant'.}

Dr N.   That's right. I've only just felt it. [Laughter] I mean if that isn't useful . . . .

E.B.   He only began to realise how it was.

Dr I.   So surely that was where the work achieved?

Dr N.   Yes, a new horizon really.

E.B.   But for me it's a surprise to find your acceptance of her as she is really. I don't know whether you accept her as much now as you did half an hour ago?

Dr N.   I don't think I do actually. [Laughter] It is quite a thing – and in a sense the way that we've leant on each other – that is the thing that stops anything happening. And that last time all we did was lean on each other again instead of actually standing back and looking at things in a different way.

E.B. I would have thought looking at things and talking about them is a long way away. She'll give you other body symptoms, and you'll have to understand what she is telling you through what she does with her body.

The atmosphere in the group had been open and relaxed enough to allow the presenting doctor not to be embarrassed about forgetting the sex of the child, while allowing the members of the group to wonder why he did not know, and not be critical. In turn this allowed the doctor to entertain other ideas about his patient and feel annoyed at her, particularly about the note, despite his declaration that he 'would do anything she wanted'. He told the group he had been deeply disappointed by her decision to 'become a civil servant', which he saw as self-destructive. Until the group discussion his gratitude to her for not dying had hidden his negative feelings about her, disabling him professionally. When the doctor gets in touch with what he hides from himself he can then perhaps respond more appropriately. This is facilitated not only by the comments of the group members but also by the working environment which needs stable and clearly defined boundaries.

The stability of the external boundary is provided by the same group of doctors meeting in the same place for the same length of time each week, with the same leader, and keeping interruptions and changes to a minimum. There are also important internal boundaries. Members should not expect personal therapy. In the foregoing case of Aurora it would have been inappropriate to focus attention on the doctor's personal experience of mothering. This is not to say that the doctor's personal experience has no effect on his professional behaviour but that it is his private concern. The boundaries here are delicate and of course are often touched upon (see Chapter 6) but crossing them is not encouraged. This is quite often incomprehensible to those who have no experience of Balint groups, especially if they have been in some sort of therapy themselves. This proscription is seen as a defence. The truth is that 'the therapy' lies elsewhere, in training the doctor to listen and to see more clearly within the sphere of a professional relationship. The object is not to reconstruct the doctors but to help them accept themselves and use their capacities to the best advantage.[1] The psychoanalyst can help to throw light on this process but the general practitioners are the only ones who can find out what works for them in their own setting.

Our group was interested in studying changes: in the patient, the doctor, their relationship and in the doctor's working method. Quite quickly what we called surprises – a class of change – became the focus of our work. A surprise gives a sharp focus on a point in time in the doctor–patient relationship, so that what comes before it and what follows are different and can be examined.

There were three elements to the data we collected. Each week the seminar was tape-recorded; this was our basic data. However, tape-recorded data is relatively inaccessible and time consuming to review, therefore each meeting was transcribed. This not only made our data more manageable, but it also gave it a different perspective than that gained by listening to the tape itself. However, it must be noted that there is no easy convention to describe the para-verbal components of discussion, such as the tone of voice, the pace of the discussion, grunts, ahs, ers and ums, etc, all of which help to describe the atmosphere and mood of the group. Without these cues, misunderstandings can more easily arise. The final element of our data was a report, written up by a different member of the group each week. From the beginning, we adopted a summary sheet which was rather informal compared to those used in previous groups.[2] This approach sat well with our general philosophy of encouraging a personal viewpoint, but we had to be careful about this because while we expected and worked with a bias in the doctors' views of their patients, we wished to be accurate in recording what the group said about a case. Therefore, each summary was available for the group at the beginning of the next meeting when its accuracy was rigorously discussed, matters of fact and different viewpoints were clarified, and changes were made where appropriate.

A good illustration of the relationship between these three elements of our data was given when Dr J. presented the death of Mrs Miller at our sixty-third meeting. By chance that week we had two reports of the seminar, one by Dr J. herself and one by Dr N.; there were important differences in emphasis and meaning between them that generated discussion, making us return to the original recording to try and resolve the differences.

Mrs Miller had been first presented by Dr J. at our eighth meeting. She was from Holland, a seventy-two-year-old who had been a patient in a neighbouring practice until about three years previously when she had been removed from its list because she had been too demanding. However, her husband, a man of military bearing, had stayed with the original practice. The patient was large, overweight and wheel-chair bound after a stroke sixteen years ago. She had a very personal and often burdensome relationship with Dr J., who did not like the husband. During the year previously, Mrs Miller had lost her sight and the doctor had read letters to her from relatives in Holland because she shared her mother tongue which the husband could not speak.

Here are the two reports about Dr J.'s last presentation to the group. They only refer to ten minutes of an hour and three-quarters seminar in which we also discussed the previous week's report, our research and a new case.

Dr J.'s report
At long last Mrs Miller died in August while Janet was on holiday. On her return Janet called at the home; to her relief Mr M. was not there. Social Services sent her a list of items and requests they needed for Mr M. which Janet curtly sent back, reminding them that he was not on the practice list. However, Janet is still hoping to meet up with Mr Miller.

Dr N.'s report
Mrs Miller has died. Social Services contacted Janet about Mr Miller; was this with his, Mr M's, knowledge or prompting? Janet enjoyed writing back that she was not his GP. She then thought of visiting and did so – but Mr Miller was not in!

Still curious to see him – 'Is he really grieving? Did he really love her?'
Enid: 'Even the Millers are difficult to part with.'

Comparison of the two reports was inevitable, because of the discrepancies – was she *hoping* or was she *curious* to see Mr Miller? Dr N. was prompted to listen to the tape of this discussion, which at that time was untranscribed. He produced his own transcription for the group to read at the beginning of the meeting. This is the first two and a half minutes of it:

Dr J.   I'll just tell you that Mrs Miller has died. She in fact died while I was away . . . . so as far as I hear from the hospital she died peacefully . . . . just went to sleep and didn't wake up . . . . Um I had some communication from Social Services . . . about Mr Miller saying well for . . . . sakes do something because he needs this, he needs that, he needs his hearing aid altered and he needs all sorts of other things, and I just have curtly written to them – I'm terribly sorry but Mr Miller was not our patient, my patient, nor anyone else's in this partnership, could you please get on to his GP.

Dr L.   You enjoyed that. [Laughter all round] Ooh! you did.

Dr J.   I was half thinking of going to see him, and I did go to see him. [Dr D.: You did?] And he wasn't in.

Dr D.   You really have, you have ended with a flourish haven't you?

Dr J.   Um . . . . . and I haven't been since and I feel bad about it really.

E.B.   You feel bad about it?

Dr J.   I think I should see him.

E.B.   Gosh! What shall we do with the girl? [Laughter]

Dr J.   I was delighted when I heard that she had died, I was very relieved,
        I was . . . . she deserved it, but I/

Dr L.   How old was she, I forget?

Dr J.   She would be 73 now.

E.B.   But she'd been ill for . . . . ?

Dr J.   Oh 16 years. [Mm, Mm from several] Yes.

E.B.   But you feel guilty, because you haven't been to see him.

Dr J.   I don't feel guilty. I owe it to myself to go and square it out with him,
        face to face now; then I won't have that awful feeling about the sick
        woman there in the background about whom I couldn't do a thing or/

Dr L.   What do you want to sort out? I'm sorry you totally lose me?

Dr J.   I want to see him, if he's grieving if he's um . . . See I was never sure
        whether he loved her or whether he really hated her and/

Dr L.   You're curious.

Dr J.   Yes, I am curious.

Dr D.   Janet just wants to find out something doesn't she?

Dr J.   I just want to/

Dr H.   For our benefit?

Dr D.   {Together} No! For her own benefit.

and

Dr L.

Dr J.   I can't send you {i.e. Dr H.} there now, can I?

Dr H.   Well I don't have any contact with [mumbles].

Dr J.   I just thought, I would go, but I haven't been/

Dr H.   You could/

E.B.   You went, and he was out/

Dr H.   Go as a friend of the family.

E.B.   What did you feel when he was out when you went?

Dr J.   Relieved. [Laughter all round]

It had been particularly interesting to have two reports about the same
meeting, especially as one was made by the presenting doctor and considering how difficult it was for her to be clear about her own feelings.
Nevertheless, the other reporter also had problems in being precise about
what happened. Reducing a ten-minute discussion to a few sentences is
almost impossible. Notwithstanding that, making such reports obliged us to
define our observations and allowed us to review their validity the
following week, after metaphorically stepping back from the proceedings.

Enid Balint suggested in one of the early seminars that the focus of our
work, in remaining with the doctor–patient relationship, was like an apple

suspended in the middle of the group; each member had a different view of the apple but what they saw as a group added up to a whole. The work was about putting together different complementary, individual views. This process produces changes of view amongst the members of the group, and gives the patient an opportunity to see himself from another angle. The work is not about cutting into the apple so that the 'real' trouble can be exposed. If cutting is needed, then 'surgical' help can be enlisted or the doctor can do it himself. It is easy to withdraw to 'surgery' if one cannot face observing any more! But finding out exactly what is at the core of the apple does not necessarily help the patient.

Let us look at another case. Keeping the image of the apple in mind, and knowing that each reader will be struck by different aspects of the case, this is how Dr I. summarised Dr R.'s presentation of Ann Shipman (discussed in Chapters 3 and 4):

Had been in the practice all her life, but was rarely seen until four and half years ago when she began to complain of menstrual irregularity and pain. Within the past year a female trainee had given her the pill for the irregularity. Ruth saw her for the first time recently, since when she has attended about four times. Ruth found her an attractive girl with long blonde hair, but able to slip into the patient's seat without being noticed – in sharp contrast to the attention she received when she got there. She presented with persistent epigastric pain unrelieved by antacid, and Ruth knew that father and uncle had duodenal ulcers. She arranged a barium meal, which was negative.

Her parents separated four years ago (when her symptoms commenced), and she lives with her dad who acts as housekeeper. He recognised that her pain was probably due to her nerves but was getting worried nevertheless.

Having got the X-ray out of the way, Ruth got her to discuss her problems at home. She told her that she loved both her parents and couldn't stand the way they hated each other. They are now divorcing but her feelings about this were not discussed.

Ruth noticed how she always came at 9 a.m. and asked in a motherly way whether she got into trouble at school for being late. Ann triumphantly told her she merely showed the teacher her appointment card and all was well.

In the discussion that followed the group 'viewed the apple' from several directions.

E.B.   She chose to see you. She asked?

Dr R. She {with a light laugh} saw me. As I say, it's not clear why she saw me. I mean, my trainee, who she'd been seeing before, left in November.

Dr N. And was male or female?

Dr R. Female. But I don't know why she picked me.

Dr H. You made a comment that someone said it was possibly stress induced?

Dr G. Her father/

Dr R. Her father had said/

Dr H. About her?

Dr R. Yes.

Dr H. [Mumbles]

Dr R. No! No, she just reported.

Dr H. Let . . . . . I find myself backing off her and looking more intently at pathological causes even though it's very likely.

Dr J. That's why Ruth did a barium meal.

Dr H. I don't know why you did that? Is it because they say stress you are trying to . . . . . .

Dr B. Sorry, maybe you're going on with that. My idea was to do with her being a very unforthcoming patient for you and that was a way of looking inside her.

Dr I. Or forthcoming! How unforthcoming? You'd expect a fifteen year old/

Dr B. I'm not saying . . . . She seemed to be for Ruth, for Ruth a surprisingly unforthcoming patient. Maybe she's not really you know, but that it was Ruth who expected more from her. But I was struck by the initial description that she seems to hide herself. She's in there before you had noticed, and some idea around that seemed to relate to how she gets involved in her parental fighting; that she tries to hide her feelings about how much she hates it all; until that one moment, quite charged, she told you. She doesn't express her feelings very openly. She has to absorb all her parents' comings and goings, but she has to get ill with them rather than have a good yell.

Dr R. I think that is very clear how they use her in that way. She said at her mum's she used to answer back and try and defend her dad; but now she doesn't. She just sits and waits until it is over.

Dr I. I have a lot of hope for this girl. She is not acting inappropriately for a fifteen-year-old girl with all the stresses and strains. Somehow she has found herself with Ruth, who I am sure is going to see her through the next few difficult years. She seems fairly well together.

Dr R. I was very impressed with this girl. I think I brought it not because it's a particular surprise/

E.B. I think that comment of hers was wasn't it?

Dr R. It was that comment of hers, but also/

Dr I.   What? That she can't stand, she hates/

Dr R.   That she can't stand the way they hate each other.

Dr I.   I almost wrote down {Dr I. is writing the report for this meeting} that she can't 'stomach'. I wonder whether she did use the word stomach?

Dr R.   I can't remember the exact words.

Dr J.   It's pretty unusual that a child should go with the father.

Dr I.   She was only eleven.

Dr H.   It's unusual too not to side with one or other. [Dr R.: Yes.] She can't stand or she can't stomach.

Dr J.   So did she elect to go with father or was it her agreement with the parents? . . . . are there any women about?

Dr R.   I haven't gone into that yet.

E.B.   I don't think it's really relevant, but still.

Dr R.   The feeling I get is that mother has got another man.

Dr H.   Did she use the word hate?

Dr H.   Because I heard you saying she hates them both. As if she's saying a curse on both your houses.

E.B.   She can't bear how they hate each other.

Dr H.   Yes I know.

Dr I.   She *loves* them both.

Dr H.   Sorry, what?

Dr R.   She can't stand how they hate each other, and then said later how she loves them both. She can't stand/

Dr H.   What I heard was, 'I hate the way they can't stand each other'. But she didn't say that? Is she really upset? Does she want a smack on the bottom? What does she want to achieve?

Dr J.   Or was she so good about it that she wanted to bring them back together? And now she sees it's not working and she's going to have a lot of belly aches.

E.B.   It is very difficult to stomach hatred, isn't it? [Several agree] The way that Ruth spoke about it so vehemently. I felt it was how the patient spoke about it. You slightly raised your voice and said, 'I really can't stand this hatred'. [Dr R.: Mm] I don't know whether the patient actually said that, but this quiet fair-haired girl suddenly exploded that she couldn't stand something. Am I inventing this?

Dr R.   No. I think that is exactly how she comes across . . . . . it was a mini-explosion. It was a bit unexpected. Obviously there was something there and in a sense I was very glad that it surfaced like that, but it was a bit of a surprise. But it also relates to . . . the reason I've brought it is because we've been thinking about questions of technique . . . . I . . . . The question of the barium meal and things was on my mind a bit as well.

After this most of the group found it quite difficult to 'view the apple' from a variety of positions; they congregated in one place and spent a lot of time worrying about the propriety of referring Ann for a barium meal. Almost all but the leader became so strongly identified with the doctor that they were only able to connect with the doctor's professional discomfort, which then spread on to issues of prescribing the pill to minors, and the doctor's realisation that she had over-identified with Ann.

During the course of our work we were interested in discovering connections and our discussions were often like associations around whatever meaning such connections might have for the patient. These were a prelude and an initial tuning for what the patient had to say at the next visit. In Ann's case, even though her father could see the connection between her stomach pain and her nerves, it was the patient and her doctor discovering it together that mattered. Dr R. needed to discuss her patient with the group to see what had happened more clearly. When Ann saw her doctor the next week she said her stomach ache had gone. She seemed much more open, smiling, and Dr R. felt that 'she had come much more out of the furniture and was very much with me in the room'. Ann told her doctor a lot and was very forthcoming. She and her doctor appeared to be engaging in an appropriate and important dialogue.

In this chapter we have described the chosen method of our group, which assumes that the 'observer-error' is a dimension of every consultation. This can then be examined in the seminar to help the doctor adjust his viewpoint. The same phenomenon needs to be challenged rather than accepted when it affects the assumptions made by the group. The method combines training with research. Our research hypothesis was that a 'surprise' indicated a change in the doctor–patient relationship, and that as a result, new connections might be made, and that what happened before and afterwards was open to study; the meaning of each surprise, however, remains subjective.

This hypothesis has the merit of paying attention to a tension that exists in general practice between the need to be able to generalise research findings and the wish to make sense of the experience of individuals. It accepts the unexpected as something useful rather than a complication. If the reader can accept the difference in focus of our enquiry from that of more traditional medical research, a great strength emerges – our method of enquiry is not dissociated from the method of our daily work. They serve to accentuate each other.

NOTES

1   See 'The limited though considerable change in personality' (Balint 1957: 301).
2   Previous research groups have used a 'form' to report their cases on. Some groups even made their initial presentation of the patient to the group from the form, which they had completed before the meeting. The 'form' was first developed in 1949 by Michael and Enid Balint at the Family Discussion Bureau. Its evolution is described elsewhere (Courtenay 1968:10).

6 The observer-error

Indeed, the necessity of considering the interaction between the measuring instruments and the object under investigation in atomic mechanics exhibits a close analogy to the peculiar difficulties in psychological analysis arising from the fact that the mental content is invariably altered when the attention is concentrated on any special feature of it.

(Bohr 1933:459)

This chapter extends the previous discussion and defines more closely what the group meant by 'observer-error'. It also touches again on how the group managed personal revelations.

The belief in the value of the subjective touches on fundamental and paradoxical ideas about reality. Is 'reality' the world out there, something external, or does it predominantly gain its appearance from within the mind and is therefore internal? These two views can be presented as contradictions. However, objective and subjective 'realities' coexist and are not mutually exclusive. They have an important dynamic relationship; each illuminates the other. In the present rather over-rational climate of medical thinking this relationship between subjective and objective is easily overlooked. If too great an emphasis is given to the apparently 'real' external world, ironically, it leads to further distortion, the very thing such an approach seeks to avoid.

As with subjective and objective, so within the subjective there is a dynamic relationship between reason and feeling. Reason has for a long time been considered the crown of humankind's endeavour, and, unfortunately, feelings are often wrongly equated with the irrational. This is misleading and is often used as a justification for the disregard of feelings in the name of reason. Reason and feelings are not opposites; they coexist. They influence each other. Denying feelings does not prevent them affecting reason; it simply hides their action and obscures their effect. Paying attention to feelings is the first step in taking the observer-error seriously. This is particularly difficult as feelings are often communicated without either party being fully aware of them.

Pursuing the idea of the observer-error with the help of general scientific concepts allows a new perspective on the doctor–patient relationship to emerge. The original Balint emphasis on this relationship has degenerated into a cliché, which now means little more than 'getting on well' with the patient – a 'good' or 'bad' doctor–patient relationship. Surprises informed the group directly about the doctor–patient relationship and made it more accessible to consider and investigate. The following example demonstrates these points and their relevance to the work of general practice.

Mrs Angela Denton and Wayne (first mentioned in Chapter 1 and fully described in Part IV – The Booklet) gave the doctor a surprise in the consulting room and he had a further one in the seminar discussion. These two surprises were associated with each other. You will recall that Mrs Denton had brought her son Wayne, aged eleven, believing he was choosing to be deaf to her. After the doctor had demonstrated to his own satisfaction that the boy did have a genuine high-tone deafness, he took the boy's side. While this obviously pleased Wayne, the doctor neglected the effect it had on his mother, until she surprised him with her parting remark, which praised him, by saying to the student how wonderful her doctor was. The doctor told the group, 'I realised instantly that I had put both feet right in it and had not paid attention to her but had only been looking at Wayne'. He recognised in her praise a cry for attention and felt chastened and guilty for ignoring her.

Why had the doctor interpreted her undoubted compliment in this way? He said that, when he saw the look on her face and heard the compliment, he sensed that it was mixed with some criticism. The student did not see it that way. This is one aspect of what is referred to as the 'observer-error'; no two individuals report the same event identically, each has their own perspective. The student heard only the patient's words and agreed with them. The doctor, however, was left with a feeling of discomfort arising from the sense that he had got something wrong. Neither the doctor nor the student were necessarily correct, but the doctor's perception meant that he was open to look again, which turned out to be very helpful to both mother and son. We will now follow this case further to show how and why this was.

Mrs Denton's remark was delivered as everyone stood up at the end of the consultation and it 'left all four of them dancing a jig in the middle of the consulting room'. All her doctor could say was, 'Bring him back in a week's time'. She dutifully did and the doctor, demonstrating that the hearing test was unchanged, sent Wayne into the waiting room to read a comic while he talked with Mrs Denton. He told the group about it like this:

Dr L. I said to her, 'I wasn't paying attention to you last week, I was only paying attention to Wayne.' At which stage she broke down in floods of tears and she didn't sort of say yes or no in actual words. So then I gave her a tissue and let her cry a bit. And she kept saying, 'I didn't want to do this, I didn't want to do this.' And I asked, 'You didn't want to do what?' and she said, 'Cry!'

She went on to say how awful it was being a one-parent family and how she was absolutely driven to be disciplinarian. The doctor then went on:

Dr L. 'Well you obviously thought that I was accusing you of being beastly to Wayne last week', and she said, 'Well I suppose that is certainly how I felt that you proved me to be, as beastly as that'.

And we had a bit more tears. Then I got her to verbalise how she saw the problem she had, and what of course she is trying to do is be two parents rather than one. She told me about the various minor problems of getting him to do homework, getting him to school, getting him to do what she wanted him to do. She felt she was always on at him even though she knew it was counterproductive. She did not know any other way of behaving. So then I turned round and said, 'Well it is possible just to be the mother and not be so disciplinarian, if you feel that is what mothers should be.' She was silent for quite some time before she said, 'I'm not sure I could do it, I'm not sure. I just feel that I have got to make him do his homework and other things, and the problem is that his father does have access to him and this always leaves him in a very distressed state. I really don't know how to handle it.'

The doctor accepted this and made an appointment for her to come back to discuss things further. He imagined he might see mother and son in a joint interview next time and try to help them move out of this rather fixed state. However, when they returned two weeks later it was quite obvious that they had already had a talk together and the 'joint' interview had gone on at home with the doctor only present in spirit. Even though Wayne looked well and was smiling, he had another problem. Apparently he had been getting short of breath when playing sports for about six months. The doctor demonstrated an exercise-induced asthma which responded to treatment with an inhaler.

In this case the doctor picked up Mrs Denton's complaint that she had not been heard whilst she was genuinely complimenting him to the student. Many of us would either have delighted in the compliment or have been embarrassed by it and so missed the irony and the opportunity to use it. In hearing it, the doctor understood Mrs Denton and gave her the opportunity to return. He then talked with her alone but at her pace and stayed with what she brought. This in turn enabled her to deal with Wayne more appropriately at home. Mother and son were both encouraged by this to return to talk about a disabling condition which Wayne had had for six months. Perhaps he had until then kept it from his mother or she had not wanted to hear about it or trouble the doctor with it. The important point was that they were both able to behave more freely.

As the group's discussion progressed another explanation emerged for why the doctor ignored Mrs Denton during the consultation. He surprised himself by recalling, out of the blue, how as a child he was thought to be swinging the lead, when an episode of abdominal pain had not been taken seriously until his appendix perforated. This was an experience which would have had an undoubted influence on his subsequent view of the world, and would contribute to the 'personal dimension' of his observation. Personal dimension is a polite term for bias and most scientists would attempt to exclude it from their observations. This may be legitimate if objectivity is at a premium, or where vast amounts of information are received and criteria must be found to disregard some. In this work, the doctor's being, his perceptions and gaps in them, are his guide. The doctor acts as an instrument of measurement. Dr L.'s instrument, influenced through a missed appendicitis that burst, would inevitably tend to pick up over sensitively on a boy with a real hearing loss accused by his mother of 'choosing' to be deaf to her.

Errors that surround observation in any setting fall into two main classes: those that are random and those that arise from an ascribed cause. Errors of known cause arise from three basic elements – the observer, the instrument and the object observed – but also the interactions between the three of them.

Mrs Denton in the example had an effect on her doctor, when she came to see him with her son to talk about how she felt he was choosing not to hear her. In some way the doctor quite quickly picked up a particular slant on their relationship and only paid attention to Wayne. The doctor was shocked into looking at the situation again not only by the remark she made but also by an awareness that the direction of his attention could be subtly influenced by the resonances of the relationship in front of him. The doctor in his turn, however, had an effect on what he observed when he sided with Wayne emotionally – sorry for the son and dismissive of the mother. This is a clear example of the observer having an effect on what he looks at and being reciprocally affected by what he sees. That each affected the other in an important way is obvious with hindsight. At the time it was only the remark and the surprise that it caused him which informed the doctor that this was so; without the surprise nothing would have been obvious.

The interaction between observer and observed is a universal phenomenon, towards which every branch of science has a characteristic attitude. The analytic chemist challenges it and attempts to avoid all errors. The behavioural scientist, however, accepts rather than challenges it, and in trying to understand and make use of it has evolved the concept of the 'participant-observer'. Physicians adopt an attitude somewhere between these two, at times challenging and rejecting 'errors' while at others accepting and working with them. Doctors often have a prejudice against the concept of the participant-observer within medicine. This attitude is driven by two concerns: one with accuracy and the other with objectivity. The former may result in the extremely accurate description of trivia – Polanyi makes the point that 'accuracy is not of itself valuable to science' (Polanyi 1958:136).[1] The latter misunderstands the attitude of the basic sciences, in which as long ago as the 1920s, Niels Bohr, the Danish physicist, evolved his principle of complementarity.[2] This recognised that when measuring the behaviour of atoms it was impossible to measure particle and wave properties simultaneously. Two different views were therefore obtained of the behaviour of an atomic unit, and neither was more nor less objective than the other. Bohr considered that each view was complementary to the other and that taken together they presented a fuller picture than when each was taken alone. Later in his life he explained his concept to a much wider audience, believing it could throw light on to a wide range of human experience where man was both participant and observer. Each could give a different but complementary view to the other, which when taken together offered a fuller picture than either could alone.

The doctor, in the example cited, participated fully while he took Wayne's side but this stopped him observing until he was shocked by the mother's praise. His instant recognition that he 'had put both feet right in it' was like a massive deflection on an internal meter. He achieved this by engaging both aspects of himself; the participant engaged his feelings and enabled the deflection to register; the observer saw it and interpreted its meaning.[3] The doctor cannot pay attention to these two functions simultaneously but only in sequence. Each gives a different but complementary view to the other and widens the doctor's concept of his work with the patient.

Whenever doctors use their feelings like this, as a personal internal meter, they open themselves to the kinds of error to which any instrument is prone. What troubles the patient may be obscured if the doctor picks up other 'sounds'. These may arise from inside the doctor–patient interaction or they may be extraneous. Wayne's doctor was subjected to the 'sound' of his ruptured appendix which led him to side with Wayne, and so the signal from the mother was masked. Feelings like this, which are important elements of the doctor's instrument, may generate internal disturbances in the doctor which are indistinguishable from what troubles the patient. These disturbances by analogy with unwanted sound are called 'noise'. They can arise just as easily either within the patient – so that the signal sent out is mixed with unwanted 'noise' at source – or, much less commonly, from entirely outside the system of doctor and patient. An example of this extraneous 'noise', technically called interference, is given by the student sitting in with Wayne's doctor, who possibly encouraged the doctor to pay more attention to the 'proper' clinical problem of deafness. The doctor quite easily and naturally isolated himself from this interference by ensuring that no student was present when he reviewed Mrs Denton.

Just as these two issues, noise and interference, are ubiquitous in the world of instrumental measurement, so they are in the doctor's consulting room. Provided the ratio between signal and either noise or interference is good, it offers the group a chance to amplify even quite a small signal and the seminar becomes the 'laboratory' where this takes place. It is achieved by the group 'listening' carefully to all aspects of the presenting doctor's narrative. Quite often a signal given out by the patient, barely perceived by the doctor at the time or dismissed as unimportant, is amplified by a remark in the group and the doctor then responds by remembering a whole host of things, which suddenly seem to make sense, giving a new perspective on the patient.

The case of Mrs Sandra Morgan, already discussed in Chapters 3 and 4, demonstrates how both elements, 'interference' and 'noise', caused her doctor problems and obscured the signal. He started telling the seminar about her like this:

Dr L.   I have the greatest difficulty in actually remembering her name . . . I had to ring the surgery to find out her name . . . but it's not just her name . . . it's all sorts of things . . . Her name is Mrs Sandra Morgan and she is forty-three in a fortnight's time!

Such recall and precision surprised the group. The doctor went on to say that the patient had come first about two years previously and had seen the trainee for oral contraception. Her boyfriend was getting a divorce and already had two children while she had none. Three months later she first saw Dr L., this time with a missed period, not having used her contraception, explaining that at forty plus she was anxious about her fertility. As soon as her boyfriend's divorce came through, she wanted to marry him and have a family. Her pregnancy test was negative.

She did not come to see the doctor for another nine months, which was shortly after she had married. Her period was again late and once more her pregnancy test was negative. She was disappointed, declaring a sense of pressure to get pregnant. The doctor gave her a temperature chart and referred her to the local gynaecologist who had an interest in infertility. He saw her within a month and quickly established that her hormone profile and post-coital test seemed fine. However, the patient just as quickly referred herself to a private clinic, where they gave her a different and pessimistic view of her hormone levels, which her doctor followed only through the correspondence from the clinic.

Three months later she returned to her doctor asking for referral back to the first gynaecologist. Her doctor, wanting to understand, asked her to explain her request. She could not. He asked her if she wanted the first gynaecologist to test her hormones again. She said that was not it, more that she was forty-three in a fortnight's time. The doctor told her he understood this and rehearsed the referral letter he would send. However, this brought an unexpected response:

Dr L. She then backed off saying, 'Oh it doesn't matter, perhaps I'm silly to want to see him'. It was a most peculiar feeling. I had had difficulty in getting close and, when I thought I had got it, it disappeared . . . . that's the sort of thing that is happening with this woman. She is always disappearing into some mist so the only thing I remember is her birthday.

The doctor was conscious of fertility occupying the foreground of their relationship and this seemed to prevent him hearing anything else. This 'noise' seemed to originate inside the patient, and perhaps hid other things that were troubling her. The group also felt that there was some noise inside the doctor which was preventing him receiving the patient's signal. He had behaved quite unlike himself. It was most unusual that this doctor had not found out more about his patient and what sort of state she was in. This was perhaps also a consequence of interference, created by the patient when she referred herself to the second gynaecologist. Referrals anyway have a tendency to produce 'interference'. For Sandra Morgan's doctor it was as if the interference and the noise resonated in him to such a degree that he could hear nothing else. What troubled the patient remained obscure. In the discussion the group was unable to amplify what the patient was trying to say. This was frustrating for them. They pushed the doctor harder. No new understanding of the patient emerged but the doctor recalled that his own mother was forty-four years old when he was born!

At this point, before continuing the exploration of the observer-error, it is worth diverting to look at what the group did when the doctor made this personal revelation. They did not attempt to explore what this meant for the doctor but instead were released to ponder some of the mixed feelings Sandra Morgan might have about a late pregnancy, which as yet she had been unable to talk to her doctor about. As Dr B. put it, 'The difficulty is her desperate two-mindedness isn't it? I mean, it's easier to be either encouraging [or not] – it's the desperate two-mindedness.' More importantly the group understood that the doctor's insight about his mother's age and the realisation of how this might be affecting him offered him the chance to quieten the noise in order to pick up more clearly whatever the patient wanted to say next time.

The doctor's personal revelation was a measure of how much the group was pressing him. Their attempt to amplify a signal from the patient which the doctor had not heard simply increased the noise inside the doctor until it burst out of him. The group was no longer a simple sound laboratory, interpreting signals from the patient, but had become more of a 'workshop' examining the doctor's instrument. The way a group responds to the noises it hears inside a doctor helps to define a Balint group. It would have been easy for the group to continue examining the doctor's feelings about his own mother as if he were the patient. This would be legitimate in a group offering personal therapy but it is not the remit of a Balint seminar which meets to examine the doctor–patient relationship and to describe what is going on in general practice; an exacting task, easily avoided if the group is distracted into personal therapy.

It should be emphasised here that although the amplification of the doctor's internal noise is not the focus of the group's attention, it is a common consequence of its attempt to amplify an obscure signal from the patient. Usually the noise in the doctor can be clearly heard by the group long before the doctor perceives it. The group may then be tempted to point it out and try to discover its significance, in an attempt to re-fashion and improve the doctor's instrument. It is better for the doctor to be left to hear the instrumental noise only if he wishes. If you only have a crystal-set, complaining about the quality of reception instead of listening to the broadcast is rather pointless and distracts attention from the message! Another case from a different doctor illustrates some of these points.

Jill Norman (discussed in Chapter 3) was a rather seductive looking, black haired, twenty-three-year-old, but her doctor, a woman, always thought of her as more like a fifteen year old. She was difficult, an epileptic with multiple behaviour problems, an IQ of about 80 and a very thick record file. She had first come to her doctor about four years previously when she moved with her family from Liverpool after being raped by her half-brother, who was now in prison. The patient's mother was a binge drinker and avoided the doctor. The father, a quiet merchant seaman, who had probably held things together, had suddenly died about a year ago from a heart attack. A few months after this Jill got herself pregnant and concealed it from the family and her day-centre staff until she was eighteen weeks pregnant. She then came to see her doctor asking, 'Will they take it away?' The day-centre staff, who had already brought her to the doctor for contraception, were set on a termination and arranged it directly with the hospital, much to the doctor's fury, while the doctor was away on leave. After this Jill attended her doctor frequently with symptoms of bleeding, abdominal pain and nausea. This went on for about six months. The doctor then described to the group how, two days previously when she last saw Jill, she felt as if struck by a thunderbolt because she realised that she had never asked Jill how she felt about her termination. Jill had then graphically articulated her feelings of loss.

It emerged in the group discussion which followed that at about the time of Jill's termination the doctor had herself suffered from a miscarriage although she was now securely pregnant once more. The doctor had only made this connection during the group discussion and suffered another thunderbolt in realising how her own instrument had been unavailable to signals about lost pregnancies. It was as if the noise level in the doctor about this topic had been so loud she had turned off all reception to it. Although members of the group were aware that the doctor had miscarried they had not pointed this out but had let her make the connection. However, they were interested in how the doctor would use her insight and imagined that now she had re-opened channels about lost pregnancies she might hear only this and ignore Jill's other losses. In other words, they felt that the doctor's 'resolution' of what was troubling Jill might have been concluded too soon. 'Error' of this sort could effectively prevent Jill talking to her doctor about other feelings of loss.

The power of resolution, in terms of the instrumental analogy, is the ability to distinguish between two readings that lie close together. For Jill's doctor it would not only signify her ability to distinguish the origin of a feeling – was it in Jill or herself? – but also the ability to distinguish between similar but different feelings – particular feelings about mis-carriage or a more general sense of loss.

Although both cases – Sandra Morgan and Jill – involved explicit personal revelations by the doctors, they serve here to illustrate the constant phenomenon that everything doctors perceive about their patients is re-ceived through the myriad of variations and characteristics of their own experience. It is unusual for a group member to overcome a block, as Jill's doctor did, quite so explicitly during the course of the seminar. Paradoxic-ally, the understanding it generates may force the doctor into a premature resolution of observation which is often not helpful to the patient. For-tunately, it is much more common for the doctor to be left puzzled, like Sandra Morgan's doctor was, with a feeling that things are not quite right. This is helpful because he knows that his resolution is low, he has checked it with the group, and then pays more attention to the patient at the next consultation. Knowing that one does not know allows the doctor to become more open and receptive.

This chapter has described what the group meant by 'observer-error' using a classification derived from the theory of measurement to show the increased varieties of bias the doctor is open to when he allows himself to become a participant-observer. We hope that these ideas give a wider perspective on the doctor–patient relationship and show how as a phenomenon it can be examined and understood for the patient's benefit.

NOTES

1   Polanyi tells the story told by E. Warburg of Friedrich Kohlrausch, the German physicist, who offered to measure accurately the speed of water running in the gutter; 'meaning that scientists must be able to recognise what is manifestly trivial, just as what is manifestly false' (Polanyi 1958:136).
2   Rosenfeld says about complementarity: '. . . no formal definition of it can be found in Bohr's writings . . . ' (Rosenfeld 1963:10). The *Britannica* definition of the Principle of Complementarity is that it 'implies the impossibility of any sharp separation between the behaviour of atomic objects and the interaction with the measuring instruments . . .' (*Britannica* 1988).
3   Enid Balint first talked about this concept in a paper she gave at Montreux in 1984, which was included in the book *While I'm Here, Doctor* (Elder & Samuel 1987). She describes how the doctor must 'first identify [with someone or something] and then he must withdraw from that identification and become an objective professional observer again. The identification must have a biphasic structure.' She also makes the point that 'the doctor must be able to respond correctly and without too much delay'.

7   Surprisability

... Now, coughing, the patient expects the unjudged lie: 'Your symptoms are familiar and benign' – someone to be cheerfully sure, to
transform tremblings, gigantic unease, by naming like a pet some small
disease with a known aetiology, certain cure.

(Dannie Abse, 'The Doctor', from *Way out in the Centre*)

It is often said that doctors should treat their patients as individuals. What
does this mean? How possible is it? Consider for a moment the number and
variety of different people a doctor might see during the course of a single
working day, and the subtlety of their individual needs. The phrase may
usually mean, simply, that patients should be treated with respect and not
as objects of the diagnostic and therapeutic process. But, more specifically,
what hope do we have of responding to the individual needs of our patients
in any single consultation? Or in the terms of the last chapter, fine tuning
our powers of resolution? How well *can* we hope to know our patients? It
is easy to collect information about them but that is different and often not
helpful. Our ability to relate to people accurately is anyway inextricably
connected with our own concerns. Does it follow that if we understand
these better, or at least monitor them more closely during the course of our
work, that our patients will have a better chance of being treated as
individuals?

In the last book to be published by a group of Balint doctors, *While I'm
Here, Doctor* (Elder & Samuel 1987), the cases described were almost all
heavy or burdening to their doctors. The authors of that book became
interested in these burdensome feelings and made a study of the changes
that sometimes occur to transform them, or at least temporarily lighten the
load. These patients have recently been well described as 'heartsink'
patients (O'Dowd 1988). Michael Courtenay had earlier described how the
difficult patient cannot be considered without consideration of the
'difficult' doctor; that the feelings engendered arise from the relationship

between the two (Courtenay & Hare 1978). In this chapter we want to start by making a clear distinction between this sense of 'heartsink', or dread, which all doctors will necessarily have towards a small group of their patients, and a more generalised feeling of irritation, which may not be so necessary, and which may lead a doctor to feel dissatisfied at the end of a particular surgery in which he has not seen any 'heartsink' patients.

Most doctors will be familiar, at the start of a surgery, with the feeling of wanting to 'get through' their list of patients. The list of names seems to represent a series of potential pitfalls which the doctor must somehow or other navigate successfully without getting too badly bogged down or knocked off course. But by the end of some surgeries the doctor may feel enlivened by his contact with the patients he has seen while at the end of others he may feel drained and dissatisfied. It often seems that when we most seek to conserve our energy, perhaps seeking to 'get through' the list of patients quickly that day, that we are likely to end up feeling drained; but, conversely, when we approach our work with a less hurried and more open-minded attitude that we are more likely to finish feeling satisfied, and quite possibly, quicker too! It does seem that by trying to save time, foreclosing on our consultations before they have properly started, we may waste time and energy.

Early on in the life of our group we became interested in unexpected events occurring in consultations, events which we later called 'surprises'. An earlier chapter (Chapter 1) has described some of the many different forces that may lead a doctor to be surprised during the course of his work. Potentially surprising events are likely to be occurring all the time. If a doctor is capable of surprise when he is practising medicine, then he is likely to be alert. Considering the immense variation of diseases and people that general practitioners come across, it is rather surprising that we are not more often surprised! As the work of the group progressed, the doctors in the group were faced with this question. Why were we not more often surprised? Was it that we were not sufficiently open to register the shifts and changes, contradictions and disparities around us, being too intent to 'get on' with a single-track view and not wanting it disturbed? Or was it that we were squeezing our contacts with patients through a medical 'sieve' to limit our personal exposure to what otherwise might be too much or too painful? There are great pressures on doctors to 'know' things. Do we screen out discordant observations or unexpected experiences in order to comfort ourselves with the illusion that we 'know' our patients? Or was it that we were not noticing because our attention was focused too much on 'the patient', and not enough on our own reactions and on the relationship?

It does seem that surprises are enlivening and yet are also resisted. Surprisability implies an openness in the doctor's mind, and a willingness to learn. Without that openness how can the doctor be surprised? If the doctor is operating in a single-track fashion, he will tend not to notice any new information or unexpected feelings, and fit all observations into the mould of his pre-existing ideas about the patient.

At the beginning of a consultation with a patient who the doctor has seen a few times before, he starts with a general feeling of what he knows about the patient – not only what he may or may not know about the medical history and family circumstances, but a vague contour in his mind of the patient as a person. Such an impression will be based on many things, amongst which will be the doctor's past experience of the person as a patient. The doctor may have a strong tendency to fit whatever happens during this consultation into the mould made by past impressions. At the outset of such a consultation, there may not be much willingness in the doctor's mind for an alternative view of the patient. However, if he now approaches the same consultation, this time only loosely aware of what has gone before and not too strongly attached to that view, holding what he knows about the patient against a stronger sense of what is unknown, then there may be more willingness, a larger space in his mind – with a slightly negative pressure – surrounding his previous view of the patient, into which a new perception of the patient might spring, surprising him.

We often tend to cling to the status quo, seeking familiarity but deadened by it. New experiences seem to be avoided, but, paradoxically, bring our work to life. Being conservative is sterile both for the doctor and the patient, and the doctor is likely to end his surgery feeling irritated. The patient will not have been able to bring anything new about how he is feeling to the attention of the doctor; and the doctor will not have learnt anything new about the patient as an individual or what the patient needs from him. Of course, in many consultations, if the doctor is functioning in his normal mode it is possible for the patient to get what he needs, in which case both will be sufficiently satisfied with the outcome. The question is how surprisable are we when the patient needs more, or is trying to communicate something that we have not yet registered? How sensitive is the surprisometer when the terrain has changed? Do we strenuously ignore all the signals because we feel we 'know' what the patient wants in the (false) belief that this will save us time and energy? It may be that when a patient is held at arm's length in this way, and his distress not accepted, that it is particularly exhausting for the doctor, as well as unsatisfactory for the patient.

Doctors are trained to be unflappable, or imperturbable, even unshockable. Almost all the emphasis in medical education is on the acquisition of knowledge. Good science involves a sound sense of what is not known, of the unknown, as well as a healthy scepticism about what is thought to be known. Doctors are not renowned for this. Doctors carry great burdens and responsibilities and their own need for security may lead them to keep within areas where they feel most sure of their ground. As anxiety levels increase, so will this tendency, as both the patient and the doctor will increasingly try to rely on the doctor's knowledge. That knowledge appears to be a life-raft, particularly when life is at its most threatening.

In most cultures the doctor is also expected to have knowledge of a different kind. He is expected to have travelled in frightening places before and to be a comforting companion in places of great unease. Nothing should surprise the doctor. He has seen babies born and people die. However strange the complaint, the doctor is expected to encompass it and to have some idea of 'what's for the best'. All general practitioners will recognise the patient who gives three sentences of vague symptomatology and then pauses, 'What could it be, doctor?' How tempting for the doctor, pressed for time, to say 'such and such' and hope the matter ends there!

What does seem important is for the doctor to be able to hold a balance in his mind, of what is known to him about his patient and what is unknown. It is in the space held open by the awareness of what is not known that lies the room for new observations, for movement and change, for something surprising or creative to happen.

This freedom to think is often not available to the doctor at the time when he is with a patient. It often seems as though the doctor's airwaves are jammed, by powerful forces that render him unable to function in his normal mode. These powerful effects on the doctor's performance lie quite outside the doctor's control, and may originate in the patient or may arise from within the doctor. One of the doctors in the group reported a patient with whom he had felt 'paralysed' in just such a way.

Miss Jean Carter, recounted in Chapter 1, was a young woman in her twenties, who came to see her doctor, complaining of feeling low and of early waking. The patient was the youngest of three children, and her mother had been one of the most seriously ill patients that the doctor could remember. Mrs Carter had suffered from a manic-depressive illness which had lasted over ten years. The doctor had been very involved in her care and told the group that her life had 'hung like a thread'. She had been stabilised on lithium and had been well for the last three years, but the memory of her long illness was still painful to the doctor. The daughter Jean ascribed her own state to a change in her conditions at work. The doctor described being 'in a cleft stick' feeling unable to mention anything suggestive of her mother's illness to her, but also wanting to assess the severity of her depression, and whether this was the onset of a similar illness in the daughter. To the other doctors in the group it seemed pretty clear that there was a big difference between mother and daughter. They were less worried about the daughter, and thought that it would not be difficult or damaging for her to tell the doctor about some of her thoughts and memories of her mother's illness. The doctor, however, felt quite unable to do this in a way that was completely uncharacteristic of his usual style. He felt immobilised. It became clear during the discussion that, for the doctor involved, it had been as though the patient's mother had been sitting there and not the daughter at all. 'I couldn't take another Pamela', he said. The distress of the mother's illness with which the doctor had had to grapple over a period of ten years, and which had included him having to support the hospital psychiatrists when they were at their wit's end in knowing how to manage her, was still active enough, by association, to paralyse him when confronted by her daughter. It appeared to be more painful for the doctor than the daughter. The daughter's illness might well have been related to her mother's but not in such a direct way as the doctor imagined.

Considering the nature of medical work, it is likely that we are often paralysed by patients in this way. As in this case, the difficulty may be associated with someone who is just off-stage, but often it arises through past dealings with the same patient. The doctor may be puzzled by a feeling of being locked in a particular track, and not being free to move in his usual way. In this kind of case, if the doctor is surprised at all (other than by his immobility), it will be during the group discussion. Whatever has been pinning him down may be released during the discussion as the doctor listens to the other group members' reactions. He returns from a painful identification to being a more objective observer again.

Enid Balint has described what she termed a 'biphasic structure' to the identification that occurs between a doctor and his patients. Once an observer has identified himself with someone or something, he will find it difficult to feel objectively about that person or thing again. So he must first identify and then he must withdraw from that identification and become an objective professional observer again. The identification must have a biphasic structure (Balint 1984). It may be that as the doctor leaves such an identification he is likely to be surprised; the withdrawal may suddenly enable him to 'see' where he has been! The change, however, may not always be back to being an objective observer, but sometimes into a different identification with the patient; professional work is a series of such movements. Often the patient does not need the doctor to make such a change; but if he does, either because what he needs from the doctor has changed or because the two have never been sufficiently on the right wavelength, then the doctor may make the change successfully or not. He may be prevented from doing so by pain associated with his relationship with that patient, or he may be free enough emotionally to make such a movement. It is in the movement from one phase to another, if he is sufficiently observant of his own reactions, that he is likely to be surprised. What seems to matter most is whether he is free to move when the patient needs him to do so.

One of the doctors in the group reported a recent contact with a patient he had known for thirty years. He had felt 'profoundly depressed' after seeing her, possibly more than he could ever remember being after seeing a patient. He had started the day feeling fine. 'It just sat on me all day.' The case was of Mrs Susan Towle, earlier recounted in Chapters 1 and 3, who had been recently widowed. The doctor had seen her twice since her husband's death. Mr Towle had died suddenly in the street whilst out shopping with Susan. He did not like doctors much and had only seen the presenting doctor rarely. The doctor was unable to give a death certificate and a coroner's post-mortem was carried out. Susan herself came from Lancashire, but was described as a typical Claphamite. She had been the first female out of forty-three pregnancies! She had a deep voice and was 'tremendously sort of dismissive of men, over the years, with a dry sense of humour, very wonderful sort of little comments, very sharp, I always felt very warm towards her'. Susan had brought presents back for the doctor from all over the world. The doctor had worked closely with her at times of earlier distress in her life. There had been virtually no sexual life between her and her husband, who had become totally disinterested in her after the birth of their only child, a daughter. The doctor had always felt that she and her husband were not particularly close.

On this occasion Susan came to see the doctor bearing her husband's death certificate. She had seen his body after the coroner's post-mortem had been carried out. 'It was awful. They had cut his head open and he looked an absolute mess.' She was obviously extremely distressed, no longer covering her feelings in her usual manner, and the doctor was profoundly affected by her grief. 'Not that she said very much, we have got a sort of language over the years, and it just flowed into me, and utterly depressed me.' The doctor felt that he had never known her and said that he 'had obviously totally misjudged the depth of her emotional life, for a very long period of time'. He was profoundly affected by this feeling.

This case stimulated a great deal of thought in the group, and during the discussion many different aspects of it were considered. The doctor had felt quite out of touch with her. He could not reconcile his previous knowledge of her, the jokey, dismissive, Clapham bus conductress, with the Susan looking at her husband in his coffin. Her remark was out of character as well, neither ironic nor dismissive, 'he was a complete mess with his head cut open'. Did the patient that the doctor thought he had known exist at all? Was this a new Susan? Or one that the doctor had never known? Or that she had never allowed him to know? Or that she had never known herself before? Had she always loved her husband, despite the difficulties in their marriage, much more deeply than the doctor had ever realised? Or that she had ever allowed him to realise? Or had she herself been overwhelmed with a feeling of remorse, looking at her husband's damaged head, of sorrow for their damaged relationship? Perhaps she felt something very similar to what the doctor was later to feel, 'I never really knew him', and sorrow for the undone years. Had some of the doctor's feelings come from guilt at not being able to provide the death certificate himself, and therefore to spare Susan this ordeal? Was Susan feeling guilty and was the doctor picking this up? Susan had suddenly become a womanly woman after years of being a manly woman, the 'forty-fourth male' in her family. There was an abrupt change and their former relationship was suddenly felt by the doctor to be dead. There was a strong sense of suddenly being without defences, being laid bare, in the raw. There was no doubt that during this reported consultation the doctor had closely identified with the patient and she had communicated something very powerfully to him.

In this consultation with Susan the doctor was surprised (shocked would be a better word) at the moment when he suddenly saw a new Susan and at the same moment, by contrast, saw his old working relationship with her thrown into relief. In a sense all observation occurs by the perception of contrasts: one sight or sound, one thought or feeling, set against another. The observer, in this case the doctor, must be sufficiently alert and open to register such changes, and contradictions.

The doctor arrived at the next consultation with no preconceptions. After the sudden dissolution of past patterns, he neither knew whom he was to meet nor what to expect. His strength was his defencelessness. He was in a heightened state of unknowing, perhaps a particularly good starting point for any contact with a patient. 'I had no clear plan in my mind.' After a few initial exchanges in which Susan seemed to be like her normal self, the doctor referred back to their last meeting. 'You know Susan, I've known you for thirty years, and I felt as though I had never known you at all.' The tears rolled down her cheeks. The doctor sat there with her. The tears washed away any doubt that he could help her. They were for herself, for her husband, but perhaps particularly for the years of banter which had prevented her from knowing and being known, and which she had used to hide her emotional needs. 'All my life I've had to look after other people and I want to be looked after now.' There is not a hint of jokiness. It is one of the clearest statements that Susan may have ever made about what she feels she needs. It comes after the doctor's utterly unambiguous statement of his own feelings which reaches into the heart of their relationship.

The doctor was now able to find out how she envisaged her future and to express his willingness to care for her. There was a question of early retirement which could have been granted by the union man at the garage. 'If I'd slept with him I'd have got my early retirement but I've never been one to sleep around.' The doctor had said, 'I am perfectly prepared to carry sick benefit as long as it lasts, if that is what you want'.

The group was initially hugely relieved and moved by this report. Susan now seemed sad, appropriately sad, 'neither ill nor depressed or covering it up'. It was remarked that if the doctor had not referred back to the previous week, this consultation might have carried on in the old vein. There was discussion about how much Susan herself had really changed, and what might be the outcome of the changed relationship with her doctor. One group member thought it had 'enabled her to actually grow from this experience, she can both be her jolly self and look back on this terrible unhappiness. She's changed, she's not the same person she was.' The doctor himself commented, 'I felt we left with a new relationship, though very new and untried, but very little to do with our previous one'. If there was a new relationship, was it different in quality to the relationships she had had in the past? Others were more cautious, thinking that more could be seen about the doctor's change than could be seen of Susan. Again the question arises, how well do we really know our patients? How good at knowing any patients are we? By jumping to conclusions about changes, we were perhaps trying to deny our surprising unfamiliarity with this patient, and denying another great source of surprises, our ignorance of outcome. Had the patient ever had a relationship that wasn't either jolly or depressed?

It can be seen in this discussion that just as the doctor has to withdraw from his identification with the patient in order to remain observant and professionally useful to his patient, so the group has to work on its own identifications in the same way, with the help of the leader. If the doctor (or the group to a certain extent) cannot withdraw fast enough, then he will be limited in his usefulness to the patient (or in the case of the group, to the doctor). These changes are very difficult to observe and need to be followed carefully to see how useful they are to the patient.

If we now return to the group discussion, one member began to express her anxiety about Susan's future. 'I am still terribly worried for her because you are actively encouraging her to retire . . . ' Had the doctor's own expectations of what he could repair for Susan of the past become too great? If this was so, could there be a threat to Susan's autonomy, arising out of the doctor's strong feeling for her predicament? He can use his under-standing of what has happened to help construct a useful professional relationship for her, but he cannot repair the past. ' . . . the problem is this woman is quite tough, she will cope I think but the doctor has got to put up with being a semi-success. You look after her, you will see that she does not have to go back to work, but you cannot supply the years, twenty years or whatever it is.'

This case can be seen to be progressing, with the doctor being surprisable in the first place and receiving the impact of changes that the patient undergoes; identifying with them, and then allowing himself to be modified in such a way that he can be more useful to the patient as a result. There is an ebb and flow, to and fro. First he is open to the new communication, then, at the right time, not immediately, he uses it, touching directly the root of the patient's distress. Both of these phases are necessary for healing to take place.

We hope it can be seen clearly through the description of this case that useful professional work in our setting proceeds through these different phases of identification and change, and that at many different points during these phases the doctor may be 'surprised'. To register surprise, the doctor must not only be open to the complexity of his work, but also be observant of the detail of his own reactions to what he notices and not brush them aside as extraneous.

Part III
The wider context

8 Narrative research and scientific method

> At the same time I realised that such myths may be developed and became testable; that historically speaking all – or very nearly all – scientific theories originate from myths . . . I thus felt that if a theory is found to be non-scientific or 'metaphysical' (as we might say), it is not thereby found to be unimportant, or insignificant, or 'meaningless', or 'nonsensical'. But it cannot claim to be backed by empirical evidence in the scientific sense – although it may easily be, in some genetic sense, the result of observations.
>
> (Popper 1963:38)

Alongside the group work on the presentation, analysis and follow-up of cases which forms the bulk of this report, we spent a considerable time discussing the nature of our group method, the choice of focus for our research, and the difficulties of data analysis. We also spent time considering other questions which concerned us as much. In what way is our group work useful? Is it scientific? How does it fit into current ideas about research in general practice?

At first sight these may seem to be the inevitable anxieties of the parents of a cherished research project. At the heart of our questioning, though, ran a feeling of disquiet about the nature of much research in general practice. We were concerned about the current concentration on quantitative methodology almost to the exclusion of narrative and qualitative studies, and the implication this carries for the values assigned to the different methods involved.

It is generally seen that the central activity of general practice happens within the consultation. 'The strength of general practice lies in the privileged loneliness of the consulting room' (Bain 1991). What kind of attention is accorded to this? How are we to study it? How are we to evaluate what doctors perceive their patients are saying to them and what the doctors' own contribution is to the outcome of their work together? Of course, there has been research on the consultation but there has not been much which includes the doctors' attitudes and blind spots as part of the material.

It is an essential part of the Balint method to stay close in beside the doctor. Inevitably, this takes us to the borderline between story telling and the discipline of science. Many of the questions which a group of this sort asks are not those which can be subject to the null hypothesis. They may be too closely tied to an individual case, or related to a set of phenomena such as emotions and thoughts which are evanescent and subject to a multitude of influences, and so in that sense cannot become scientific questions. Nevertheless, the descriptive narrative may be of immense value. Detailed observation may illuminate the stages of a complex interaction; and as with stories in other parts of life, allows readers and other observers to experiment by imaginatively trying things out for themselves. The narrative allows us to recognise and observe our feelings and experiment with solutions.

At other points we would argue that the research questions generated within the group do fulfil the discipline required of the experimental method in science. The group method is a process that helps the doctor to heighten his powers of observation and enlarge his view of what has been brought to the consultation (both by the doctor and the patient) and so encourages him to think critically about his range of responses. Here is something that can be framed as a question with a possible answer. Is this method – of enabling doctors to make observations and to recognise their own observer-error – of value to themselves in their everyday work with patients? Much more difficult, but ultimately more important questions are: Do those doctors who are trained in this way help their patients differently? Are they more effective, or are they perhaps a hindrance?

In the next two sections, material from the transcripts of our discussions will be used to chart our progress through the question of method – is it story or science? – and then to show how we settled for looking at change and surprise as a focus for the group research. Finally, we will look at some of our discussion on the value of this sort of research both for the individuals within the group and for those who read the reports.

OUR METHOD – STORY OR SCIENCE?

We had extensive discussions in our attempt to focus clearly on the nature of our group research method. In the early stages some of us were uncertain whether we did indeed have a method, and whether what we were doing could properly be called research!

Dr O.   . . . I think we are not in the business, of in our kind of work and research, of making a hypothesis and testing it. That is knowing what you want to know. I think we really are in a position of not knowing what we do not know. But knowing that there is a problem there.

E.B.   Aren't you likely to throw up a hypothesis?

Dr O.   Oh yes, but I think that the whole philosophy of this kind of research is that it is *action research*, that is the hypothesis stems out of the actual work, it does not precede it, and I think that is absolutely crucial, so I am very comfortable with the idea of researching a theme, like a theme of what we might call three people or five people. The frame we take is the encounter between the doctor and the patients and we look out from that. Then I think we must be in the business of making hypotheses. Those hypotheses can eventually surface.

The idea of doing action research similar to field work done by sociologists or anthropologists was an appealing approach. After all the doctors were in the difficult position of being both presenters of cases, the subjects for much of the group discussion, and the researchers who formulated the final report.

Qualitative research, whatever the discipline of origin, has a set of methodological characteristics which our group shared. The enquiry tends to be naturalistic, aiming to understand what is going on without disturbing it too much, and in this sense it is not experimental. The data is based on interviews and observations. It seeks out meaning, and is always conscious of the context in which it is carried out. It is often said to be 'grounded' or 'inductive' research rather than hypothetico-deductive. The idea is that the observer attempts to minimise preconceptions brought to the data, and to allow the models or hypotheses about what is going on to emerge from the observations rather than be imposed on the observations from the start.

The discussions in our group recapitulated many of the themes about the nature of knowledge and reasoning which have been debated over centuries. The nature of our own data meant that we rarely needed to be reminded about the importance of the observer as instrument, and the contribution he makes to the data as it becomes recorded. 'Facts cannot be observed as facts except in virtue of the conceptions which the observer himself unconsciously supplies' (Whewell 1840). But we struggled with the tension inherent in the difficulty of paying attention to a broad mass of complex data without overt prejudice, and the acceptance that we can only make observations through a narrow frame of our own concepts.

Dr N.   I would make a plea that we should not focus on what we want to look at, until we've actually presented a case or two. I feel that if we

> look too soon and try and focus too soon . . . it's going to make it
> difficult to work.

. . .

Dr B. I think this goes back to the discussion about training versus research and it's extremely difficult isn't it? If you start off with some
kind of research focus that then becomes a sieve through which
people bring certain kinds of cases which is maybe how things start,
and maybe that's what people want to maintain. But it also has a
very inhibiting effect because you begin to think 'is this a proper
case for the group'. The idea of doing random case analysis is a way
of getting back to just, you know, anything that is going on isn't it?

. . .

Dr H. Random cases are fine, but the basis for this selection has to be
made explicit. Everyone has got their own private reason for
bringing a case and we can't do research on that basis.

This reminder, that in every act of the observer/researcher there is already
a set of ideas, caused us continual difficulties. How do we start to choose
our topic, how do we start to choose our research tools and language, do
they indeed emerge from the presented cases, or do we start with the ideas
and hypotheses already?

Dr O. . . . Now what I suppose I am hoping for, Henry, rather than
predicting, is if you look at these situations, these clinical situations,
we will begin to develop a language and some conceptual tools for
looking at the problems and perhaps finding out ways of unblocking
them.

Dr H. What is it that you do not know?

Dr O. I, – How can I know that I do not know?

Dr H. Well, if you do not even know that, how can you even predicate the
research? . . . .

Dr O. I'll answer that in a moment.

It would appear from this exchange that the case for our group using the
hypothetico-deductive approach won the day at this point. But the argument continued *sotto voce* through several other transcripts. Why was this?
There might be two reasons for this. Firstly because the hypotheses which
members brought to the group were inchoate, and took a lot of time and
modification by group discussion to clarify. So it appeared that the ideas
emerged late, but examination of the transcripts showed that the concepts
of observer-error, surprisability and examining change in the doctor rather
than the patient emerged early in the life of the group. Other hypotheses
which were proposed early on were not used at all. The second reason that

this became an important theme was related to our desire to persuade people that our method is part of the scientific enterprise and that this way of working is of value to doctors and patients.

To demonstrate this we would need to show that there are benefits for patients, and to show it in a way that would conform to the methods of science – that is, to be stated as a hypothesis which can be submitted to refutation.

Dr O. I think that if what we want to do is honest and valid, then we ought to be able to get money (a grant), providing we do not pretend we are going to be able to do something we are not able to do. I think for me the dilemma that I see – and it came up earlier on – we could do a piece of research, which would just be another piece of natural history; we could work at what it is, but you made the point Enid, you wanted more than that. We want to know whether our interventions are good or what counts as a good intervention or a worthwhile one and that really becomes experimental science.

But for our group at present, this was wishful thinking, beyond us in complexity. In the company of eminent scientists we needed to look somewhere less daunting for the time being:

Like other amateurs Koestler finds it difficult to understand why scientists seem so often to shirk the study of really fundamental or challenging problems . . . he wonders why the 'genetics of behaviour' should still be 'uncharted territory' . . . the real reason is so much simpler; the problem is very, very difficult. Goodness knows how it is to be got at. It may be outflanked or it may yield to attrition, but probably not to direct assault. If politics is the art of the possible, research is surely the art of the soluble. Both are immensely practical minded affairs.

(Medawar 1967)

This caused a mood of depression within the group. We all desperately wanted to find acceptable ways, in addition to our case material, of demonstrating that our work was good for patients. We toyed briefly with the idea of using a method of verification. What if we only look at what we see as successes amongst our narrative work with patients?

Dr H. Now let's accept it is an article of faith to have this group discussion. Whether it heightens awareness or whether it sorts out our individual complexities – it's helpful, but how is it helpful?

. . .

Dr H. I should like to suggest that this could give us a focus for our study or research . . . instead of teaching each other to suck eggs, why don't we employ what's so obviously manifest that somehow we know – but what we don't know is *how* we know. And if we could explore the intimacies of the case we would learn a lot more about how we sometimes, unerringly, seem to be on the right track . . . So in other words, instead of the reformists' zeal, I think we should be there as learners . . . .

Fortunately, the trap set by the idea of using only confirmatory evidence as an acceptable scientific method did not seduce us for long. The insistent outside world broke in again, asking inconvenient questions, and reminding us that if we want to speak in the language of science we have to limit our questions to those which can be challenged by the methods of science.

Dr H.   But it wouldn't cut any ice outside. They'd want to know 'Well, how do you know this?' and 'Why was this case reported?' 'What about the others that weren't?'

THE OBSERVER, ERRORS AND SURPRISES

The constant presence of quite justified criticism, voiced from both inside and outside the group, helped us to stop looking, for the time being, at trying to show how this work was good for patients and to begin to concentrate on the doctors. That's not to say we don't believe it's good for patients, we do, and those who read the case histories will see doctors attending to their patients with sensitivity. Some of the cases seem to illustrate clear changes for the patient.

In shifting attention to the doctor we were not just seeing the doctor as an instrument, someone who exhibits an 'apostolic function' or who is 'prescribable', important though these effects are. We were trying to ask about the doctors' 'mechanism' and what influence the group had upon that.

Dr O.   This is slightly off the point but it is about the research . . . I've been looking at video-taped consultations – the Pendleton approach (Pendleton *et al.* 1984) – and contrasting that with our approach. But it seems to me (that) in that difference there is something very important . . . .

Dr L.   It's the difference of the spirit and the letter. It's very difficult to delineate.

Dr O.   But in there somewhere is our research I think.

Dr R.   I think it is related to what Nick's been talking about.

E.B.   Sorry I didn't . . . .

Dr R.   I think it is related to the kind of things Nick was talking about. The observer-error, and the influence the observer has, which gets quite lost if we are just looking at behaviour.

E.B. Which if we are honest about we can, we have got very good access to examining it. If we've got the courage to examine that we can examine it.

Dr L. Yes, if our personal meters are mis-calibrated, I mean, our poor patients, as well as wasting our own time, we've got to understand what we are doing.

The importance of the observer-error, and the need to have help in the form of a group, in order to clarify and amplify one's own observations, gradually became a central focus for the group.

Dr L. I mean like Gaby's case with the woman who lay down on the couch. And I, in my own case but all the cases, almost all the cases, have that element – because I feel it is not only we who must get stuck, all general practitioners must have patients who suddenly get – you know you notice something but you cannot use what you have noticed.

E.B. I think without this kind of group though, this kind of group discussion, you do not know, you do not even know what you have noticed.

The other focus for the group's work was the observation of significant changes for the doctor and the patient. Change in the doctor–patient relationship was often seen as a key therapeutic factor, but how did we recognise change? It might be manifest as a change in how we did things in the consultation, or there might be changes which remained inside the doctor's head, or there might be just inchoate partial thoughts which needed the careful persistence of the group to emerge at all.

E.B. . . . for me the importance of Nick's case was what made him change. It was something alive about the pigeons . . . . The word I suppose I pick up is . . . change, that the therapeutic thing would be changes in . . . Nick's feelings about this chap.

. . .

E.B. Because, this is my theme, which is what I'm really interested in, so I come back to over and over again – *changes* in relationships are what interest me.

. . .

Dr R. So is our aim to understand . . . the process of the changes and what they mean for the doctor–patient relationship.

Dr L. And it is the change in the doctor?

Dr R. Well, that is the only thing that is accessible to us isn't it?

Having identified the focus of our attention it began to develop into what we called surprises. These were moments of significant change which might be recognised by the doctor, but might only be identified within the group.

Dr O.   So, it is, the problem is that we don't really have any measures of what that quality is, let alone what it does, except our own feelings. We know when we have a consultation when something happened.

. . .

Dr N.   I see it actually as championing the cause of observer-error, and giving some validity to the mistakes and the confusion that happen inside the observer. How, what happens and those sorts of things, that bit of observation which I think is very valid actually. I mean it can be just as scientific as observing what is going on outside.

The importance of the group in helping to locate the surprise and to identify with the presenting doctor some of its correlates was demonstrated in the group discussions. The group must be critical and probing so that the doctor also thinks critically about the event of change and what new course is being steered with the patient. These themes have been expounded in the chapters on the observer-error and surprisability.

CONCLUSION

So then why did we work in this way? The most important reason was that the experience of working together in the group altered each of us. This way of working sensitises doctors both to what they are seeing and what they fail to see but the group can observe.

This is the training aspect of the method, and the training continues to be needed. By necessity every generation needs to re-take the same ground and to learn the same lessons for itself. It is only too easy, with or without the discipline of the group, to engage in patient contacts paying only superficial attention which is unsatisfying to both doctor and patient.

These ideas were expressed in a number of different ways.

Dr O.   . . . there is one thing I would want to see much more up front, we should be much more reflective about what our method is about, what we feel we can achieve, that is different from other methods.

Dr R.   I was thinking before I came here, that how much being here has changed me *again* in terms of how I look at particular cases.

. . .

Dr L.   How I saw it is if we ask the question, here we are noticing changes in the doctor–patient relationship what is also going to come out is this. I think the essential thing to say is that we actually become sensitised because of the way we do it . . .

. . .

Dr L. I was coming back to the old thing, the Balints always used to say that we only perceive our patients differently when they take out a hammer and hit us over the head. It seems to me, is it possible that we can actually change without their needing to take a hammer to us?

There were other aspects too. Great value was attached to some of the attributes typical of qualitative or anthropological work. We all agreed that making a story was important in the work of general practice, not only the story for documentation, but the story that helps the doctor to capture meaning and detail in his daily work. It puts flesh on the skeleton of epidemiology applied to general practice; and provides a mechanism, a model, a theory, which allows people to talk about the meanings attached to people's behaviour. And perhaps most importantly it helps us, in the creative act of story telling with patients. Not in the crude sense of covering over or making things up but in the creative sense of helping people to find their own narrative line; adjust it in the face of unexpected, painful illness; or come to terms with an initially unpromising story.

From the story that runs between the doctor and the patient may come a series of questions which can be examined further. So this sort of research may be diagnostic. It may help in formulating a series of questions accurately, or in generating ideas that can be tested in a variety of ways. In this group we have made some progress, but we are only at the start of something which could be a most fruitful view of medicine.

At present we have established that the Balint group is a research and teaching method. The doctor and the group can make a broader range of observations together than alone. This group has sharpened up the tool, and has identified changes, surprises in the doctor–patient relationship, as a focus for the Balint method.

Dr N. In some way we have to give more credibility to observer-error, and we have to grasp that the internal view of the world, and the very personal view of the world that we have, actually affects the way that we observe things. And that is as real as the real things outside us that people look at, and that in some way we have to give that a validity amongst the scientific community . . . . .

And the proper way to do that, although difficult, and in a systematic way beyond the remit of this particular group, was also clear.

Dr N. (continues) . . . . and the way that we can give that a validity is not just by looking at it, contemplating our navel, but to show that the changes that come about are to do with that bit of ourselves. But we have to relate it to our patients otherwise I think it becomes nonsense. We have (to), that's how I see it.

To do this will be challenging. It may require using the Balint method in novel ways. But the challenge is to ask in what ways we can show, in a systematic way, that this form of training and research method is useful to our patients as well as to ourselves.

I think, Socrates, as presumably you do yourself, that in this life it is either altogether beyond our powers, or at least very difficult, to attain certain knowledge about matters such as these. And yet a man would be a coward if he did not try with all his might to refute every argument about them, refusing to give up before he has worn himself out by examining them from all sides. For he must do one of two things: either he must learn, or discover, the truth about these matters, or if that is beyond his powers, he must grasp whatever human doctrine seems to him to be the best, and to offer the hardest resistance to refutation; and mounting on it as upon a raft, he must venture into danger and sail upon it through life unless he can mount on something stronger, less dangerous, and more trustworthy . . .

(Plato)

9   Drawing the threads together

Healers are hosts who patiently and carefully listen to the story of the suffering strangers. Patients are guests who rediscover their selves by telling their story to the one who offers them a place to stay. In the telling of their stories, strangers befriend not only their host but also their own past.

(Nouwen 1976)

Making sense of medicine is a challenge. Even in the hospital setting, relating scientific knowledge to patient care is very difficult, and most patients in hospital are there after the filtering process of assessment by their general practitioner. For the latter anything and everything the patient brings to the consultation must be understood. It is daunting and exciting. But it is the very stuff of Balint work. In its fifth decade a completely different situation in general practice has to be faced, on the surface anyway. Gone is the isolation. Formal training for general practice is statutory. Academic departments of general practice are countrywide. General practice literature is burgeoning. Research is fashionable. The health service is undergoing radical change. Where does the spirit of Balint blow?

Unfortunately, it is currently not a rushing mighty wind. But it was in the 1950s, when general practitioners were castrated in traditional medical terms, and despised by many specialist colleagues. In that desert were born two forces: the Balint movement and the College of General Practitioners. One was deeply committed primarily to human relationships, while the other was concerned primarily with intellectual excellence. Not, of course, that they are mutually exclusive, just that sometimes they are restless bedfellows. It could be forcefully argued that Balint thinking was a major force in those early years when the College charted the course of training for general practitioners of the future. Many of the draftsmen were Balint trained.

What were the aims established? Surely the provision of skills appropriate to the setting. The considerable though limited change in personality sought by Balint training was a side effect of learning new skills. The choices arose in considering which skills were deemed most useful, or even essential, and the means by which they were best acquired. With regard to Balint training the relevance of the involvement of psychoanalysts in the work was because their commitment to a life-long quest for personal growth and development was shared by general practitioners.

While the College commitment to continuing medical education is undoubted, the central theme was the raising of standards over the whole spectrum of general practice work, but this was mostly directed towards concerns arising from the vast field of specialist work. Various areas are on offer, from a high standard of technical care to interactional elements in interview technique, but it remains the sum of parts rather than a whole. From that standpoint Balint work is just another dish on the menu. But Balint work is a quite different kind of learning. However, because it is not recognised as such it is often ignored or even denigrated. The real difference between the Balint work approach and the main stream of academic practice is that in the former the focus is on the doctor as a person, relating to the patient as a person in distress, with the emphasis on the interaction rather than the story; in contrast, the academic approach focuses on the story and the context, and the data which can be collected by the doctor from the patient and those around him. As Pellegrino says: 'From the academic standpoint no unitary explanation or logical method can encompass the several different *reasoning* modes and several kinds of evidence acceptable in answering the different kinds of question the clinician must answer' (Pellegrino, 1979). Attention to the science of decision-making has been patchy, and has rested most firmly on an intellectual foundation paying attention to the logic of any given situation, to the tacit exclusion of the emotional factors which clearly affect almost all the decision-making processes. Yet, as Pellegrino continues, 'the academic doctor will readily agree the end of the medical encounter is essentially restoration and healing, rather than precise diagnosis or scientific truth'. Howie has stated that we must recognise that the cellular type of general practice research can only play a modest part in the development of our science (Howie 1984). He reminds us that Kuhn argues that the time to rethink the appropriateness of a framework is when it becomes progressively less able to answer the questions asked of it (Kuhn 1970). Although the early fact-gathering has been essential to the origin of many sciences, the result is usually, in Kuhn's words, 'a morass'. He states that 'No natural history can be interpreted in the absence of at least some implicit body of intertwined theoretical and methodological belief that permits selection, evaluation and criticism'.

McWhinney (1983) views medicine as in such a state of crisis; the loss of confidence, the questioning of fundamentals; the widespread interest in the philosophy of medicine. He asks what part family medicine is playing in all this? Will the result be a change of paradigm and, if so, what will the new paradigm be like? He concludes that it will pay more attention to illnesses which fall outside the traditional disease categories, and focus on the person and his relationships and environment. It will restore the doctor–patient relationship to its rightful place at the centre of medicine. Can the Balint work concept be the crucial factor in effecting the paradigm change which is so clearly necessary to the future of general practice? It would certainly enfold traditional medicine, not replace it, satisfying both Balint's and Kuhn's visions. But this can only come about if the old lamp is taken down off the dusty shelf and rubbed clean, so that once more the Balint genie will appear to show us the way to the treasure that has been lying in the darkened cave for too long now.

The members of the research group whose work has been described herein were recruited mostly from doctors with Balint work experience associated in one way or another with academic departments of general practice. This idea emanated from Enid Balint, who wanted to re-examine Balint work with colleagues who would bring an especially critical approach to the task. It also seemed that there was a feeling current among general practitioners interested in Balint work that they had somehow failed to get across what they considered the Balint message, which they considered important, to fellow general practitioners.

While the original book, *The Doctor, his Patient and the Illness* (Balint 1957), was in almost all general practice libraries, and repeatedly appeared in reference lists to all sorts of research papers, it had taken on the appearance of an important fossil, rather than a living organism. The reasons for this generated a lot of speculation. Some of it seemed associated with the eponymous dimension of the work, and there seemed a strong current of reaction against it based on a feeling that the approach was 'old hat' and no longer relevant to current general practice. Some of this reaction seemed to emanate from a distrust in British medical circles of anything to do with psychoanalysis, some of it from doctors in academic departments of general practice who seemed to be dismissive of anything that could not be counted.

In the struggle to make general practice 'respectable' again after the nadir it was probably inevitable that the research programmes of academic departments and other college members should start with straightforward counting procedures in what was virtually a virgin forest of potential data. This kind of endeavour also had the advantage of producing results which could be readily understood by the traditional hospital-based researchers. But the initial enthusiasm for the research undertaken in Balint seminars had given way to mere respect for a milestone in the history of general practice. How had this come about?

The current group was well aware that the original aim of transforming general practitioners into psychotherapists had given way to an attempt to integrate the insights from the early work with the ordinary consultation in general practice. This had led to the work described in *Six Minutes for the Patient* (Balint & Norell 1973). While the book had seemed to generate a great deal of fresh interest among general practitioners, this had evaporated, probably because its message had not been successfully transmitted. This was seen to be partly due to the expectations raised by the title, suggesting general practitioners would be shown how they could deal with their difficult cases within the time constraint imposed by the notional time of average doctor–patient contact. However, its content remained tantalisingly opaque; the magic promise of the 'flash' had not been realised, and a fresh approach to explaining Balint work seemed necessary. It might be difficult to raise a good defence against a charge that even this research had not fully faced the core problem. A fresh approach was seen to be as crucially necessary to the work of the members of the research group as to the profession as a whole. Although the group members were personally convinced that the experience of Balint work had transformed their professional lives, just how and why this was, was difficult to describe in terms which would be likely to be accepted by doctors committed to a rigorously objective approach to medical science. These appeared to be irretrievably wedded to a somewhat rigid interpretation of the hypothetico-deductive approach. In recent years the physical sciences have reinterpreted the method in important ways. Medawar had stressed that the scientist's flight of imagination in producing a hypothesis for testing was the necessary first step in the research process (Medawar 1969). It was only after the necessary flight of imaginative, mathematical thinking that modern physicists had revealed a view of the universe very far from the mechanistic models of the beginning of the century. However, this does not yet seem to have radically informed biological thinking above the level of microbiology, and that field may seem a far cry from the work of the general practitioner in his consulting room or by the patient's bedside.

Nevertheless, the experience of continued personal interaction between the sick person and the generalist is very real, even though it is always difficult to quantify. How does one 'code' the nature of the doctor–patient relationship? To give it a value on a scale from one to five, in terms of very good to poor, is to completely miss the point in Balint work terms. The relationship reveals things about the patient and the doctor as persons, and their nature affects both the way in which the patient presents the illness, and the way the doctor responds. In Balint work terms it would be possible to have a very friendly but totally unproductive doctor–patient relationship. To approach the patient's complaints as if they were separated from the personality, and to ignore the personality of the doctor entirely, is, surely, to sell the interaction short. Even consideration of just the two-person relationship is barely taking into account the wider field of the relationships of both patient and doctor which inevitably send out ripples across the vast lake of society. General practice research is in great danger of accurately measuring things of only peripheral importance. There is a need to establish what general practitioners can do which no other doctor is in a position to do!

One great obstacle to progress is the concept that feeling is somehow less valid than reason. It is a concept which dies hard. This is all the more surprising after the concept of cognitive therapy was born some twenty years ago. Now the connection between thinking and feeling seems almost obvious. The old image of the production of anxiety being a direct reflex from facing danger has to be modified by the appreciation that the urge to flee from a lion on a jungle path is mediated through the realisation, through rapid but thoughtful recognition, that the lion is a dangerous beast. Nevertheless, it must not be forgotten that feelings often govern what it is possible to think in specific circumstances. The emotional climate generated by a particular context will tend to direct the reasoning capacity into particular directions, in a way which does not always follow the strict rules of logic.

It was in this context that the group approached the problem of reviewing the ideas which had emerged from over three decades of Balint work, determined that none of them should be accorded the status of sacred cows, and determined to eschew jargon, even if it had become enshrined in the literature by Michael Balint's gift for creating a memorable phrase. The group was determined to re-observe the nature of the two-person interaction of the patient–doctor relationship, paying attention to it in as much detail as was possible for them; and being as rigorous in the discussion of the cases as they were able.

So the quest for a greater understanding of the very heart of the work of the generalist was undertaken. This was very ambitious, all the more so because there are divergent views as to what constitutes the core of general practice work. Apart from availability, continuity and the special field of practice of the generalist, the area of two- or three-person medicine appeared likely to be the most fruitful field of enquiry. The challenge was how to become fully open-minded again. A constant struggle against using a reflex response to observations had to be waged. This involved the necessity for even greater honesty, if that was possible, in the presentation of cases.

It was not that the presenting doctors were consciously trying to distort the truth, but doctors have defences just like everyone else, perhaps more so on account of the nature of their work. An attempt to be as 'defenceless' as possible proved to be a testing emotional experience. It was here that the work in the group, taking everything the doctor said 'seriously', changed. They had to accept it initially, because, after all, the doctor was there with the patient, but, at the same time, they remained sceptical of any concept that arose too simplistically out of the group discussion, while at the same time paying close attention to the doctor's feelings. It was at this point that the value of having a psychoanalyst as leader of the group was fully appreciated, because of the fact that psychoanalysts have the capacity to look at strange phenomena, even though they may not directly encounter them in their own consulting rooms, but which are difficult for a general practitioner to see because it may be too painful to do so. They are also skilled in perceiving 'connections' over long periods of time by following the material closely. The leader of the new group also contributed an aim to have a wider look at the craziness of human relationships and the uncertainties which abound in working with patients; while at the same time not attempting to reduce them to neat patterns, leaving the perspectives as wide as possible in the realisation that what one person sees from one angle cannot be seen from another's.

Such insights emanating from the psychoanalyst were rarely challenged by the general practitioner members of the group, because it was clear that they were not based on any psychoanalytic theory, but on keen observation, except perhaps in the rare instances when a dream was reported. Even when this occurred the connection between the dream material and the patient's life was plain to see, once it was pointed out by the psychoanalyst. It was the free association of ideas that allowed the connection to appear. It has to be admitted that the psychoanalyst's skill tended to be taken for granted! After quite a short time this process of the joint working of the psychoanalyst leader and the general practitioner members led to certain things emerging, with an accompanying sense of discovery. The nature of this discovery was broadly described in terms of surprises.

The surprise might be something that arose in terms of the patient presenting some new attitude or behaviour, or something much more subtle, such as the patient making a remark whose face-value disguised a much more important communication; or alternatively just wearing unusual clothes denoting an alteration in affect. Or it might be the realisation by the doctor, through the interaction within the group, of a hidden dimension of his contribution to the doctor–patient relationship. As soon as examples of these surprises emerged, it became clear that it was astonishing that doctors were not surprised more often, one way and another. Perhaps the problem lay deep in the process of medical education, one of whose implicit aims was to fashion a suit of armour for the doctor, proof against the assaults of the distress of countless sick people, so that no horror encountered could throw the doctor into confusion. The doctor must remain unshockable. But the price is high. It makes an empathic response extremely difficult, and imposes a rigidity which allows observation to range only within narrow confines. Empathic work threatens the doctor with loss of his familiar medical role. How, then, is it possible to re-discover personal responsiveness while at the same time remoulding the medical map into a more flexible form? Perhaps by allowing the doctor to remain in touch with it with a new perspective, and so be able to offer professional help that is more useful to the patient and less threatening to the doctor.

The idea of a healing relationship seems to be generally ignored in medicine although the group observed several occasions in which the doctor identified with the suffering patient, felt the pain subjectively, and was then able to stand back in a professional manner and consciously offer the patient a possible way forward through the use of the relationship.

This was often done by allowing patients to undertake self-examination of part of their accustomed functioning, and allowing them to modify it constructively in the light of the new understanding. This was done without arrogance on the part of the doctors, who realised, on the one hand, that their healing powers were strictly limited, but who, on the other hand, observed that very small changes in a person can produce amazingly large effects on the life of that individual. It seems that the unique relationship which occurs in the general practice setting informs us as to what the work is really about. The patient says *my* doctor. The doctor says *my* patient. But it is not possession or subservience. It is working together in freedom.

Part IV
The Booklet

A case: Mrs Angela Denton and her son Wayne

INTRODUCTION

This part contains nearly all the data collected by the group about Mrs Denton and her son Wayne. They were presented first at meeting No.9 and were last discussed at meeting No.69, a span of time almost equal to the duration of the group. The data consists of a mixture of transcripts and reports.

Although excerpts from transcripts of the audio tape-recordings of the group meetings have appeared throughout the book, we also wanted to present a large sample of the data on one case, so that the reader might come to a fuller understanding and judgement of the way the group worked. There are three elements in this data: transcripts of the case discussions; weekly written reports; and transcripts of the discussions about these reports. The reports were written up by a different member each week. We adopted, from the beginning, a summary sheet which was rather informal compared to those used in previous groups, reported elsewhere (Courtenay 1968:10). This sheet quickly became essential because we could not afford regular transcripts. By the time we obtained funds, and transcription became possible, we regarded our own way of summarising as indispensable and continued with it. We found that it suited us so well that it became difficult to use the more formal method of recording which had been employed routinely in previous groups. The accuracy of our reports was reviewed and discussed the following week at the beginning of the seminar. Probably the most important shortcoming of our weekly reports was that they did not prompt us to address what had been forgotten or omitted either by the presenting doctor or in the group's discussion. We attempted to redress this by adopting the more formal style of recording used in previous groups. In practice, however, such formal presentations were only forthcoming for a relatively short time.

What follows, then, is about half the transcriptions and all the reports of one case. It is one of eight cases whose data was collated by one of us (PJ) in this way in order that each of these cases could be made up into a small booklet. This has not been done before, but quickly became essential in writing up our work and handling such a massive amount of data. We particularly wished to look at the material in much finer detail than had been the custom in previous groups. Although this may present a rather daunting prospect to the reader, the authors felt that the opportunity for the case material to be studied in greater detail should not be denied.

The booklet reproduced here is about Mrs Denton, her son Wayne and Dr L. It has been modified to exclude the transcriptions of the third and subsequent follow-up presentations. The booklet is, otherwise, exactly as we used it. The sixth and final follow-up is also reported on the 'form' to illustrate this part of the method.

The following conventions have been adopted in transcribing the discussions. It is usual during the course of a lively discussion for more than one person to speak at once. Wherever this happens and when it is possible to hear what each person has said this is represented by marking the beginning and ending of each individual's statement with a forward slash like this /Blah, blah blah/. If one person interrupts another, the person interrupted has their statement terminated with a forward slash, like this /. Where in the course of one person speaking another makes intelligible interjections that do not stop the flow of the speaker these are included in square brackets like this [Dr Z.: Mm]. Often it is not possible to make out exactly what everyone has said during a lively exchange and even with good audio equipment it is sometimes impossible to be certain what a solo speaker says. Each transcription has been listened to by at least two people (the transcriber and PJ) and may have been listened to by several of the authors.

Where it is obvious that the reporting doctor is quoting what a patient said these are put into quotation marks. Curly brackets { } have been used to enclose stage directions about group behaviour which can explain what an apparently unintelligible statement meant. A series of full stops . . . . indicates a silence. The greater the number, the longer the silence. Any silences longer than five seconds are indicated inside square brackets, e.g. [7 seconds silence]

All the original transcriptions contained a lot of para-verbal noises such as ers, ums, grunts and moans, as well as 'I means' and repetitions. For the sake of readability these have been edited out of all the transcriptions that follow but these are the only omissions in the presented material.

SECTION A

First presentation: Seminar No.9 (24.1.85)

Dr L. Well, mine is Mrs Angela Denton, who is thirty-five, brought
Wayne who is the elder of the two boys, who is eleven, to me
because he appeared not to hear what she said. She thought he
wasn't as deaf as he pretended; as a deafness of the one who didn't
want to hear; and I had a student in that morning. So I examined
Wayne's ears and there was no abnormality of the eardrums at all
and he did not seem to have had a cold recently or anything like that.
No earache as such. I did a quick screen with our little pocket
audiogram and to my surprise he, in fact, did have quite a marked
loss of receptivity to high tones, medium high tones in both ears. So
that there was objective evidence that in fact he was deaf.

Mrs Denton is divorced and has custody of the two boys. The
breakdown I do not know a great deal about, except that her
husband used to use violence on her and it was this that she called a
halt to.

I can go back into her history a little bit in the sense that she used
to be a patient of mine before she was married, because her mother
was, and still is, a patient. And shortly before her marriage she
became very anxious; in fact she had about the last attack of old
fashioned hysteria, I think I have seen, probably produced by
over-breathing and that kind of thing – it was quite interesting – just
before she got married. I did not have much time then to talk to her
about it, but anyway she did get married. Her husband was then in
the RAF, and they moved out of the practice and it is only in recent
years he came out of the RAF that she came back to me as a patient
with the two boys. Now the thing is that I was .... clearly what was
being set up was that she had been annoyed with Wayne for not
listening to what she said, and I was proving that in fact he had a
genuine hearing problem and that therefore quite clearly she had
been unjustly accusing him of being psychologically deaf, although
I didn't verbalise this in any way, but it was quite clear.

I was sitting at my desk with Wayne just at the side of the desk
and she was in the chair behind. The student was on my left over my
left shoulder and after that I said, 'Well, look I will give him some
decongestant and I want him, I must do it again, do the test again to
see if we can help him, otherwise we shall have to take it further'.
As she got up, she said, Mrs Denton said, to the student, 'Dr Linden
is a marvellous doctor you know'. So I knew instantly I had put both

feet in it and I had not been looking at her but only looking at Wayne and it was a tremendous thing because there was Wayne and Angela [Laughter] and student there and me; and we were all sort of dancing a jig in the middle of the floor and I don't know what. I just could not call it back. I was in a state of total confusion. All I could say was, 'Bring him back in a week's time'. I thought we'd sort that one out then. So dutifully she brought Wayne back in a week. And we repeated the test which in fact was unchanged. Then I suggested that Wayne went into the waiting room to read a comic and I was with Angela and I said to her, 'I was not paying attention to you last week, I was only paying attention to Wayne.' At which stage she broke down in floods of tears and she didn't sort of say yes or no in actual words. So when I sort of gave her a tissue and let her cry a bit and then she kept saying, 'I didn't want to do this, I didn't want to do this' and I said, 'Didn't want to do what' and she said, 'Cry' and I said, 'Well, tell me what the crying is about' and then it came out that of course it was the situation. She is a one-parent family, she feels that she has to make sure that the boys are up to the mark, as regards going to school, doing their homework and that kind of thing and that she finds it very difficult. She knows that she may be being unjust but again she feels absolutely driven to be a disciplinarian in this kind of situation, so I said, 'Well you obviously thought that I was accusing you of being beastly with Wayne last week', and she said, 'Well I suppose that is certainly how I felt that you proved me to be, as beastly as that' and I said, 'You're worried about being as beastly as that?' and she said, 'Yes' and then she – we had a bit more tears. So I then got her to verbalise really how she saw the problem she had, and what of course she is trying to do is to be two parents, rather than one, and she told me about the various minor problems of sort of getting him to do homework, getting him to school, getting him to do what she wanted him to do, but she felt that she was always on at him. On the other hand, she feels driven . . . . . to do this, even though she knows that it is counterproductive, she does not see any other way of, of behaving. So I then turned round and said, 'Well, it is possible just to be the mother and not to be so disciplinarian, if you feel that is what mothers should be.' And she was silent for quite a little time and she said, 'I am not sure I could do it, I am not sure I could, I just, I feel that I've got to make him do his homework and the other things and the problem is that um, his father, the father does have access to him and they are always in a very distressed state after the visits, and that kind of thing and I really do not know how to handle it' and so that I said, 'Alright, well'. I made an appointment for her to come back again to discuss the thing further.

E.B.   Thank you.

Dr H. You didn't rise to the bait, or the distress because of the father's access to the child?

E.B.   Because of what? The father's?

Dr H. Access.

E.B.   Or was it that or was it her own?

Dr H. No, I wondered whether this was an invitation for a future medical certificate to say that, for her own sake there should be less frequent visits to the child.

Dr L. That certainly did not come into my mind. This has been, I knew that there had been these little problems with access for some time.

Dr H. Do they get on?

Dr L. No! They remain bad friends.

E.B.   Am I the only one listening to this who feels she is being sadistic with the boy?

Dr N. I had a fantasy that the hearing loss was not due to congestion but due to beating around the ears, I must say; and anyway you brought him back far too soon to sort that out.

E.B.   It seems she has given him a, she's been hitting him or thinks she has.

Dr H. Does your audiometry distinguish sensory defects from conduction?

Dr L. No.

E.B.   This is an interesting one because, I don't think when you said, 'You don't have to be the father!', I mean, her problem surely is she wants to biff him and he may represent the husband for all one knows, but she wants to get him and . . . .

Dr L. That's true, yes . . . .

E.B.   There is something about her distress that you were ignoring on the first occasion. I think it was, no you were not thrown out, I don't think, at all. When you did the first interview you were absolutely right. You had to test his hearing, what else could you do?

Dr L. Um.

E.B.   But she was distressed.

Dr L. That is true.

Dr R. Can/

Dr H. It was the way he announced the findings . . . . like I do sometimes when I say, 'You poor thing, it is terrible, follicular tonsillitis, no wonder he is vomiting, no wonder he's not eating well, no wonder he stays awake all night'. And that could be wounding if the

	mother brought the child along, as a sort of 'all in the mind' sort of thing. So how did you announce what were your findings?
Dr L.	Yes, I think I did rather. I sort of said to her, well in fact I mean, 'His hearing is, isn't normal at the moment, so that I think he genuinely doesn't hear all you say'. . . . . .
Dr R.	The real turning point in the interview was when she spoke to the medical student.
Dr L.	Yes.
Dr R.	Can you explain a little more about it? Was that signalled exactly? I mean, you said that you immediately knew.
Dr H.	That you had put both feet in it.
Dr R.	How? . . . that you had put both feet in it.
Dr H.	One foot in it yes, but how both?
Dr R.	Yes, I mean I want to know where you knew so much at that point? . . . . .
E.B.	Because he already knew he was not being such a wonderful doctor, for the mother.
Dr N.	Right.
Dr L.	I don't know; in a way this has called attention to *her*, the fact that this was just under my nose, and sort of shaking hands with the student.
Dr H.	It was not sarcastic was it?
Dr L.	No, not at all, no!
Dr H.	But I am interested like Ruth. I might have just glowed with pride and missed what you did discover. How did you interpret that as a reproach?
Dr L.	Whether it was just looking at her face – which I certainly was looking at – but I immediately registered this, this as criticism rather than as praise or anyway mixed.
Dr R.	What did the medical student think?
E.B.	Thought what a jolly good doctor Leonard was.
Dr R.	Yes, I, is it something about your prior knowledge of or was it just in that interview, that has made you pick it up?
E.B.	Wouldn't you all think, if you were told you were wonderful, it was a statement that you'd blundered?
Dr H.	No.
Dr R.	Well.
Dr H.	Not when it is done to a student.
Dr R.	Depends what is going on.
Dr L.	Yes, [Laughter] I was quite clear in my own mind I had blundered in some way and I/
Dr N.	Well not, in some way, it was because it was so obvious. I mean,

when you get that sort of statement and you don't know what you have done, it's even more discomforting.

Dr L.   That's right.

Dr N.   Well, at least you knew immediately. I mean you did not quite know what to do about it, at least you came to your senses and realised what had happened.

Dr L.   I back-tracked, madly, so you know [Dr N.: Yes] What had been going on to warrant it?

Dr N.   You realised [Dr L.: Yes] what had happened. Did the third party there – the medical student – prevent you from redressing it then in some way and sending him out with a comic there and then? Which is what you could have done.

Dr L.   Yes, I think so, I think it was the presence of the medical student.

E.B.   Do you think one could have done anything there and then? I was asking myself; I believe I could not.

Dr N.   I am not sure.

Dr L.   One couldn't put it right then.

Dr H.   But hadn't you come to the end of the consultation?

Dr L.   Yes.

Dr H.   What is this? Starting all over again? What sort of world are we living in? This is not academia/

Dr N.   Because it was another patient, Henry.

Dr H.   He did not budget for another patient. [Laughter]

Dr G.   Were you surprised when you found out he was a bit deaf?

Dr L.   Yes.

Dr G.   Because I think that was the point at which you were thrown, because you suddenly had to deal with a child who was deaf.

Dr L.   I think that is true, I was surprised at how deaf he was.

Dr G.   I mean if he hadn't been deaf, I think that you probably would have turned to the mother or to the problem of – the child is not listening to the mother – he may also be deaf, and may also not be listening to the family dynamic and what is going on. I think it was then that perhaps you were thrown and you had to go off on that tack and you knew, I feel, from the beginning, that the mother came with something else.

Dr N.   And so because the rules of everything had changed so much, just like that, even if the medical student had not been there, you would have all needed to digest it. I don't know.

Dr R.   What would have happened if the medical student had not been there as a recipient of this withering comment [Laughter] about how good a doctor you were? And the lady obviously used this as a way of bringing you to your senses. She might not have been able to.

Dr J.   I do not share your anxiety about her being violent towards the boy.

	I feel she desperately wants your attention and that was one way of attracting it through the student. When her original attempt to bring attention to herself, through this alleged deafness, proved to be ill-founded as she must have had a shock herself to find him deaf.
Dr L.	Mm.
Dr J.	But also has this, she admits to trying to make them do homework, to be good, to look good, to be both parents to the boys. What is happening to her? Who looks after her? Who loves her, what has she got?
Dr L.	I, that's a lot. [Tape changes sides]
Dr J.	. . . . different feelings towards the boy. I do not get the vibration that she would be violent to them.
Dr H.	Are you suggesting, Leonard, that this was a cry for help, by her leading this boy in, with an alleged hearing loss?
Dr L.	Yes, I think.
Dr H.	Well, I am sceptical, and I think one of the things you can't decide is through the technique of recording the significant interview, when you have got a follow-up. I think a lot of our discussion is post hoc, propter hoc influenced. I simply don't know how much your report of the first is influenced, I don't say coloured, but influenced by what subsequently happened. I wonder whether as a technical matter we can encourage reports/
Dr L.	On a single/
Dr H.	At least have it registered.
Dr L.	Yes, okay. I take your point there, though I am/
E.B.	Would we have thought, if we had not known about the follow-up, that Leonard should anyway, before getting up, have said to the mother, 'This must be pretty awful for you to hear about this and you must be quite shocked'? I mean why didn't he? It's a bit odd . . . . that you never did say to the mother, she must be shocked.
Dr H.	I don't think so, in a way more treatable.
E.B.	What?
Dr H.	In a way, this could have been more treatable, than some rupturing of parent–child relationship.
E.B.	But there is a rupture in there anyway.
Dr H.	We know now.
Dr L.	Yes, I see what you mean, I can't honestly remember, I think that if I said anything now, it might be invention.
E.B.	You probably did say something.
Dr L.	I probably, yes. I think I showed that I was surprised with the audiogram . . . . . . [Noises of agreement from several]
Dr H.	Probably thought it was serious, I mean, I would have.
Dr L.	Yes . . . .

E.B. I, this, she has told you, at this second interview – I agree with that we should try to do only one – but I think she showed to me in the second, and therefore we could wonder about the third, that she is worried about being so rough with the boy. I think this is going to lead to her being rough with her husband.

Dr L. Yes.

E.B. This is just a useful . . . . trigger. I wonder if the husband was rough with that particular boy? . . . .

Dr L. I think he may have been.

Dr H. The boy is aged?

Dr L. Eleven.

Dr H. He can speak for himself.

Dr N. To whom?

Dr H. To the doctor, who is caring and insightful.

Dr L. Yes, he came in looking very sullen and certainly looked less sullen when he went out. Whether of course he saw me as the chap defending him against his/

Dr H. Well, who is the patient in the whole thing? Isn't she and I think he has got some claim?

Dr L. Yes.

Dr H. Don't you?

Dr L. But they are both patients, I mean this is what we have been talking about I mean this is what/

E.B. I think the husband is the third alright, yes. [Mumbles and laughter] Will you have to send this boy on to somebody else if his hearing does not improve or?

Dr L. Yes, I shall, I think I probably shall. I mean as Nick says I did not bring him back, I brought him back as an excuse. I think personally, I mean, one could not expect anything from mum so . . . but that was merely a quick recovery.

E.B. Yes.

Dr L. I think so.

Dr H. Provisional diagnosis?

Dr L. Beg pardon?

Dr H. Eustachian catarrh or something?

Dr L. Yes.

Dr N. Hopefully.

Dr L. Hopefully, yes. I am not at all convinced you know, I mean, I think it is surprising. [8 seconds silence]

Dr N. I mean, it does actually, in conventional medical management terms, give you time to play for things.

Dr L. Yes.

Dr N.   It does give you a chance. You have not told us when are you going to see them again, or him again?

Dr L.   The plan is that I am going to see the boy after a further three weeks but I am seeing Angela after a week.

Dr N.   Right.

Dr G.   I am quite interested in your acceptance of a physical basis of illness so quickly. Are you sure he is deaf? Because those audiogram, hearing tests are easy to fake and lots of eleven year olds are quite capable of doing it.

Dr L.   Um.

Dr G.   I am interested in you getting that result with the audiogram and so quickly going on to that.

E.B.   [And several inaudible]

Dr G.   It is just a designer fake in the audiogram and in all that he is deaf or just does not listen well and that maybe/

Dr L.   I am perfectly certain he does not listen as well as but/

Dr H.   It was the distribution wasn't it, you found a high-tone deafness?

Dr L.   Yes.

E.B.   His school has not complained about him?

Dr L.   No.

Dr N.   What sort of decibel loss was it?

Dr L.   In the 4000 frequency range. It was a 30-decibel loss so it is quite marked and I think I am quite good at telling the kids who are telling, who are saying, because in fact they cannot see what my hands are doing with the buttons on this thing. But I am not saying that he also . . . His deafness is of more than one kind.

Dr H.   My impression is that the woman is very ambitious and has to be mother and father and it occurs to me even if he had a father, wouldn't she still want to be the father? This is a point maybe. What's her appearance?

Dr L.   Um, she, I mean she is a pleasant looking woman about thirty-five, not very tall, but she is neat in physique and appearance, dresses quite well and she is one of those people who moves very quickly. She has quick movements and mannerisms. What one would term a rather anxious type of person, but that is all and she is . . . . .

Dr H.   Dresses like a female?

Dr L.   Oh yes, yes, oh absolutely yes . . . . . . I mean she certainly does not try and/

Dr H.   Does she want a man?

Dr L.   Yes. [Yawns] Oh, I think she does. I mean she has a boyfriend but not living in. [8 seconds silence]

Dr H.   The term living-in boyfriend . . . .

E.B.   Has she spoken to you about any of that in the past?

Dr L.   Not much no, it was in my mind to/

E.B.   She is anxious because she is bullying the boy, my impression is that she's probably bullying.

Dr L.   Um.

E.B.   The other one is alright is he? The older of the two?

Dr L.   He is the older of the two. The younger, there is no apparent problem but that/

E.B.   I mean this could be congenital deafness or could it be due to injury? What is the possible diagnosis if it's not catarrh?

Dr L.   I would not have thought it was due to injury, I think it would be unlikely. It is certainly not congenital deafness in the true sense, because he has been screened. He has been alright before. So this is, I think this is recent onset because he has changed to his secondary school last Autumn but er/

E.B.   If a child is anxious, would he be anxious in relation to mum, and therefore not hear? Would he be anxious for the audiogram too? Unlikely I suppose?

Dr L.   I think unlikely, much more to do with mum, I would have thought.

E.B.   Yes.

Dr L.   Yes [7 seconds silence] because in a way he has appeared, I don't know how, perhaps closer to the mum than the other, more demonstrably so than the younger boy in what I have seen. But it is a pretty, I mean, I have not seen them together very much.

Dr N.   It is interesting that I get the feeling that you want to talk to the mum and he sits outside reading the comic. I mean, I think Gaby feels that if she wants to talk to the child, then say 'Look, stop swinging the lead, I know perfectly well you've fiddled this test. It's quite easy to tell, you know, not to answer to the last two responses' . . . . .

Dr G.   Well, I feel, I am not sure if I would say it like that to him. I feel interested in the child and why he is not listening to his mother and why he is not listening at school and maybe that is creating a lot of tension at school. Perhaps that is why the mother is having to go on to him about his homework?

Dr L.   This is certainly true that he is not being good with his homework, the school have complained about his homework not about his deafness.

Dr G.   Sounds like a rather withdrawn and unhappy/

E.B.   I am worrying what does he not want to hear. Should one get at that through the child or mother?

Dr N.   I mean, it is rather an important time for him as well isn't it? He has just gone to his secondary school and he is going to make a good impression on the school? His expectations and their expectations are all being formed, and he is only through the first term and he is just coming to the second term.

E.B.   I think what is interesting for me about the whole case is that all sorts of things one would like to know about – How does he get on with his mum's living-in boyfriend? And how did he get on with his father and what did happen? Did it upset him more than the others? And so on, but this is like a questionnaire really and one must obviously not embark on it.

Dr L.   But I have some of that, certainly it was he who was, when, because in the process of divorce the father very often used to come down and make a shindi, sort of beating down the front door and it was certainly the elder, Wayne, who was the one who was most concerned and felt protective towards . . . . .

E.B.   So, if he had not had any hearing defects then one would be well away wouldn't one?

Dr L.   Yes.

Dr H.   All our comments seem to go against Leonard's orientation and discovering this technological factor and describing an organic cause. It's tantamount to saying 'That is you taken care of. Now you go out and read your comic while I get on with/'

E.B.   With mum/

Dr H.   And I am just wondering whether anyone does take offence at the traditional GP posture of dealing with the organic factors first and then seeing if there is anything left to ascribe to psycho-somatic?

Dr G.   I don't take offence at that. I do not think it is necessary to concentrate on any one or other, I think you can do both.

Dr H.   Would you have done it as a joint thing? . . . .

Dr G.   Well, I think I can understand being thrown by finding the physical thing and then getting, then pursuing that as terribly attractive; but I think um, I would hope not to be only taken in that direction but I have every sympathy with Leonard and in the way it happened. I can understand why that happened, and I think I would probably do the same thing, but I am not sure it is the best thing to do.

Dr R.   I am not sure Leonard is pursuing only one thing but when you brought up joint interviews, and the other questions of joint and whether to see mother and son together and/

Dr H.   That's what I meant by that/

Dr N.   That's what Gaby's/

Dr R.   Oh! You meant that psychological and organic together?

Dr H.   Like Leonard, I would have thought – Look, I have got to know where I stand, sensori-neural deafness, and maybe refer him, very properly, before I go on perhaps enquiring, although I said I had a claim on Leonard's attention, I believe that . . . I can't hear them both at once. Like the very first case I reported here of the woman who had carcinoma of the stomach and I abandoned all my counselling.

Dr O. I am still stuck with your reaction to her statement about you being a wonderful doctor and you decided that meant 'Hey look at me!' .
. . . . . .

Dr L. Well, that is just the way I perceived it.

Dr O. I also wonder whether there was also an element of 'Hey, stop looking at the child!' as well, that you had begun to become Wayne's and in some way this was not acceptable.

Dr L. Yes, this is quite likely and I take that and in fact she has been effective. In a way what we are saying, although Ruth has come to my defence and in fact I . . . . but this is part of the technique when you have got mother and child, how do you arrange that you see the child separately, if you see what I mean, without them saying other things to the mother, but I hope to set that up in seeing her, before I see him, because I would dearly like to see him alone, I haven't.

Dr R. I suppose a quiet hearing test might do the job?

Dr L. Well that is it, that's right yes, that is it. Yes that is the kind of thing.

E.B. And what do you do with the knowledge?

Dr L. Yes, true.

Dr N. I mean, I hear an echo coming from last week which is – 'You can only do one thing or be one thing at once'. You can only be a doctor, or you can only be a daughter and there is no way you can actually cope . . . . You can only look after one patient or you can only look after the other, which denies the reality. The whole thing is sort of/

Dr O. Messy/

Dr N. But it is only, when we become extremely anxious about what we are doing and perhaps we are doing it wrongly, we pretend that we cannot do two things at once. I mean we can look after the physical? Do we look after the emotional? We do it, together. It is only when we try and look at what we do and feel that things are going wrong that we come up with this artificial separation.

Dr G. I wanted to ask you, Henry, at what point along the course of the physical investigation into his hearing would you feel able to deal with the emotional side? When you had a diagnosis?

Dr H. What emotional side? [Laughter] What is your basis for making that diagnosis? . . . . He has failed hearing. You're ascribing that to something psychological?

Dr N.   No! Henry you are full, you are provocatively/

Dr H.   This is what you call Leonard's dilemma, this child/

Dr L.   No, my memory is actually different Henry, if I may say so, that is to say, how to handle more than one person? Which is really what triggered the whole thing and as we talk, it is quite clear to me that I must have a joint interview, because that actually would be a way forward.

E.B.   It's not quite clear to me. I think this would be an interesting, what do you do when you want to see, I mean, when two patients are there, you see the two together and you get nothing, you see them separately. How are you going to communicate, what you get?

Dr L.   Yes.

E.B.   What you hear?

Dr L.   Yes, that is right.

E.B.   I mean one way in which I do, do occasionally, is to see them separately and then together, sharing what I have got from the two separately, but you've got to get permission to do that.

Dr L.   Yes.

E.B.   It is quite a complicated, certainly very time consuming. But if you see this boy and get what he feels about it, and then you see the mother and she does not know what the boy has said.

Dr L.   I am also wondering, did I not over-identify with the boy? This has come during the discussion this afternoon from my own childhood experiences, not with deafness, with which I have had to wait many years to get, but, er, of other things, or people not paying attention to real symptoms.

E.B.   The mother has got a real symptom, she has anxiety about her aggression.

Dr L.   Yes.

E.B.   That's a real symptom.

Dr H.   This is something we have injected into Leonard now, the idea of, possibility of, reality of, violence. Now I think Leonard has to resolve that. I do not think he paid any serious attention to it before. We are talking about actual physical violence and if I were in Leonard's position, I would need to know. I would need to resolve that. I could not leave it as a vague possibility. If you have seen this woman. How can you elicit it best from her or from him?

Dr L.   Assuming I must do it you mean?

Dr H.   Yes, assuming you have it seriously.

E.B.   I would have thought, it was quite easily done at your last interview. I didn't. OK now I must, couldn't you say, 'Aren't you frightened you are too rough with him?'

Dr L. Mm.

E.B. She would have/

Dr H. But you don't see her as someone like that do you? Perhaps he does not see her as violent and rough?

E.B. I don't think he does, it's only me who does. So I'm saying it.

Dr H. But now we have introduced the idea, I mean how do you react to this?

E.B. The rough/

Dr O. When you say to someone, sorry to come back to it, 'You are a marvellous doctor' or 'He's a marvellous doctor', aren't you grossly disabling that doctor from having to talk about unpleasant nasty things? . . . . because wonderful doctors don't talk about things like that.

Dr R. Having just discovered deafness you mean?

Dr O. Yes. They certainly don't say, you know, it happened because you clouted him around the ear.

Dr J. But it just may be the inconvenience of having to go to a hospital with him and have some more time off for him from school or some more missed homework.

E.B. We'd all be distressed at hearing our boy was deaf.

Dr J. Does she work, is she? Or is she a housewife on social security?

Dr L. She is a housewife on social security.

Dr H. What did she want you to do when she came in the first time? What did she say?

Dr L. She implied that she did not think he was deaf.

Dr H. Yes, and what? How to handle it?

E.B. Tell him to pull himself together.

Dr R. Shake him and tell him to listen.

Dr L. Yes.

Dr H. So really, the announcement, however soft and matter of fact and mutual, was a denunciation.

Dr L. Yes.

Dr O. What, you, she was really saying, he has got to listen too.

Dr L. Yes.

Dr N. That is an assumption. This is something that is up for discussion in a sense. He has come along and he is not listening to what is being said and isn't this something to be discussed? There is an offer for a joint consultation which was implicit there. We are making the assumption as to what we think she wants us to do and there is perhaps a feeling in you, as there would be in me, about 'I don't want to be this sort of father to this child and therefore I don't want to discuss it. Therefore let's separate them.'

Dr L.   There was another possibility that she wanted me to be not the aggressive husband. The father who would be nice, but also get him to do is homework.

Dr N.   And that would be generated through discussing in a joint interview.

Dr L.   Yes.

Dr N.   And getting them each to feel a little bit about what? I mean I don't know.

E.B.   You see, I think she did feel Leonard was a good doctor when he has said to her, 'Look shut up, he really has got something wrong with him, he is not just being bloody'. And she was quite pleased about that but then she needed some help after hearing that, and you gave it to her a week later. She must have thought, 'God! He is good not to let me get away with my rubbish, not to be taken in by my rubbish.'

Dr R.   Right, I quite agree, because that was why I was so surprised at the way Leonard responded, and particularly/

Dr H.   Defensively/

Dr R.   Well/

Dr O.   Guiltily.

Dr L.   Right! Guiltily. [Laughter]

E.B.   I always feel that actually, isn't it right to be alerted by someone telling you, you are wonderful?

Dr O.   Yes.

Dr H.   But you are suggesting that it is to keep you quiet?

E.B.   But I think she was actually, I don't think it was just flattery, I think she was really saying something, which was, 'I am the villain and he saw it'.

Dr H.   Well, I don't think so. Now we can't look at it because there is a second interview and I cannot see anything even in retrospect. Can't see anything in that first consultation, or your description of her getting up, which would have meant that to me.

Dr L.   Meant critically you mean?

Dr H.   No, but all we have is your reaction to what she says. Did you work it out?

Dr L.   Most, very few patients tell the student how marvellous I am. It is usually my dear old ladies.

Dr H.   I am quite . . .

Dr L.   But this is, a very unusual for young girls to sort of go overboard for this thing, and I just knew that . . . . . she had expected me to pay more attention to her and less to the boy, or I mean to do with the boy – it is all wrapped up. But I had not paid, I paid lots of attention to the boy and not enough to her.

Dr H. You mean compared to what you usually do?

Dr L. No, compared to what she wanted, because her expectations of coming in as I see it, was that she needed help in handling the boy.

Dr N. The way, what the outcome has been that she has had help with herself and that what she came with and what she offered was – 'Here we are both together can we talk to you?' And you said 'No, let's have a look at the hearing'. And it is the hearing that is the problem.

Dr L. Yes.

Dr N. Er, so she still has not had that expectation met.

Dr H. That bears out what he was saying earlier, the disease can be the third party?

Dr L. The other thing of course is how much difference how much of the student contributed to my actual handling of the first part of the interview.

Dr N. Right.

Dr O. It increased your anxiety about not missing a physical diagnosis.

Dr L. Absolutely.

Dr H. But he/

Dr N. But if the student had not been there, she would not have had anybody to make that remark to and you would never have had been brought up short.

Dr O. Oh I don't know.

Dr H. No, I agree with Nick. It is common experience that while patients cannot say to your face, 'Thanks doctor, gee you are wonderful' they will say it to someone else for you to hear. Well, why isn't he listening to me? Or why isn't he listening to me? I think it was meant for you. I agree with Enid there was a compliment. Why you took it so hard I do not know?

Dr L. It wasn't so hard, I thought it was a signal. [Dr N.: Yes] You know, I thought it was a signal.

Dr H. Warning bells?

Dr L. I mean part of it was true, it had a different ring of truth in it.

Dr O. It could be.

Dr L. I knew it was true. [Laughter and mumbled conversation]

Dr O. When patients, mouth self-evident truths . . . .

Dr N. I mean the way it works then is that she means the opposite in some unconscious way. [Dr O.: Yes] Therefore, how do we link those two together? Yes, I have not been a particularly good doctor, because I have not listened to her.

E.B. And he was right, the follow-up shows it, I mean, he made that statement to himself before he did the follow-up. It is all there.

Dr L.   I actually wrote it down in the notes of the first interview before the second one. Not that I can prove that I did it.

Dr N.   What did you write in the notes, Leonard, because that would help Henry.

Dr L.   I cannot remember.

Dr H.   Resentful? . . . . . .

Dr L.   Something to do with this thing that she shook the student's hand and said what a marvellous doctor Leonard was and he must have blown something.

Dr H.   Yes.

Dr N.   When you wrote the notes, you were still a little bit unsure about what you had blown?

Dr L.   I knew I had not paid enough attention to her, that is all I know.

Dr O.   That's enough.

E.B.   Another title for this is verbal and non-verbal communication, isn't it?

Dr H.   You're a marv/

E.B.   What's said, and what we believe.

Dr H.   It sounds almost as if with the shake of the hand, of this young woman, you are the marvellous husband, the father . . . .

E.B.   Well I am thinking of Rosemary, we ought not to go on any longer. Thank you.

[Recording of this meeting finishes here. However, as the meeting was breaking up Leonard was asked what childhood experience he had had of not being listened to which he had mentioned in the discussion. He then told how his accute appendix had perforated because he was thought to be swinging the lead when he complained of tummy pain.]

Report of first presentation

Leonard then presented a case, Angela Denton, a divorced woman of thirty-five who brought her elder son, Wayne, aged eleven, to him saying he seemed to be deaf. The implication was that he wasn't listening. Leonard discovered he had a genuine high-tone deafness, and while this obviously pleased Wayne, Leonard neglected the effect that this had on Angela. Leonard had a student with him, and on leaving Angela told the student that Leonard was a wonderful doctor. Leonard immediately felt this was a signal that he had identified with Wayne rather than her, and could only say that they should return the following week. When they did, Wayne was dismissed quickly, and Angela broke down in tears over the problems of being a one-parent family, and some time spent discussing this. [Written by Dr L.[1]]

Discussion

The major issues in the discussion were:

1 Whether Angela had been physically violent to Wayne as her husband had been to her?
2 Why Leonard thought that the compliment via the student was a cry for attention?
3 What technique should be used next time – possibly a joint interview with Angela and Wayne?
4 It was a pity that a second interview had not been available from the outset.
5 Was the deafness really organic?

Note

1 This case was both presented and written up by Dr L. We tried to avoid the presenter writing the report.

SECTION B

First follow-up: Seminar No.10 (31.1.85)

Dr L. Angela Denton came back as expected; but what was *unexpected* was that she brought Wayne with her. In fact he wasn't due to see me until next week, to check his ears, and so my first surprise was that Wayne was with her. My second surprise was that Wayne looked immensely cheerful. As you remember he looked sullen and fed up and he was, his face was alive and he was obviously capable of smiling and I, I was a little bit thrown because I didn't know why he was in. He was put in the patient's chair by Angela and I sort of said, 'How's things?' and I got the impression, though I didn't actually focus on it very well, that she may have got muddled about the ears, so I repeated the hearing tests, which showed some improvement over three weeks, but also, interestingly enough, not so reliable; you remember I was tackled in the group that perhaps he was just sprucing and I in fact had to use my ploy of the silent button rather more often, though I think I, and I didn't quite understand that. Anyway, so I said, 'Well it certainly seems to be improving, we'll keep an eye on him'. I didn't feel that I wanted to go on with that.

But the interesting thing was this was a morning appointment and he was supposed to be at school, and so I looked at Angela and sort of said, you know, sort of inquiringly, without actually, I think, saying anything, I can't remember what, if I did say anything, and her first reaction to that was to say, 'I'm very sorry about last week, I realise it was PMT'. And I quote what she said as 'PMT'; that's not a horrible jargonistic thing for premenstrual tension. I mean that's what she actually said, and so I sort of looked at her rather blankly and inquiringly because I thought, my feeling was that she was . . . . that she was backing off her distress, but having said that, I had Wayne there and I didn't really know exactly how to proceed. However, I didn't have to wait because she then said, because the younger boy was going to, going off to school, she'd kept Wayne back in order to have a discussion, and that's what they'd had, a talk about everything and all her feelings about being the single parent and how she, perhaps she was being too hard on him and homework and so on; and they had virtually come to see me, after this discussion and I mean he looked quite different. They'd obviously been communicating, and she'd got it out that she'd been pushing him and why and at this particular moment obviously the relationship was not so fouled up. I asked sort of, I asked her to sort of verbalise a bit about what she'd said, and I said to Wayne you know, 'Do you feel better now?' and he said sort of, 'Yes.' So I sort of said, 'You feel that you were being got at?' and he sort of nodded and smiled at that time and so I said, 'Well it's, you realise Mum's had, has problems, just being her at home?' And he sort of nodded again. Admittedly I was leading him, but I, but he certainly was very free. It was an entirely different atmosphere. And at this point, I was completely caught again, taken entirely off guard again because at the closing of this consultation she said, 'Of course, you must never retire.' You see, I was, bringing my, after Tuesday evening I'd felt that early retirement was the only possible thing on Monday morning, actually. But I was completely thrown, I couldn't work at all with this, and I said a very odd thing, something I, it was so odd, I think I've actually had to force myself to be honest, you know and kick myself and say I mustn't, I mustn't say anything didn't happen; I said, 'You want me to be chained to the post for ever?' that was what I said and she said, 'Yes'. So I said, 'Thank you very much'. That was the end, but I was, I mean; I say it as it was.

E.B.   Well thank you.

Dr I.   Only trouble with all that, because I wasn't here last week, but reading the thing and then hearing you. It's always when she says something nice about you that she follows it up with something that she's angry with you for.

Dr L.   Mm, that's right. Mind you, when you read through the full transcript, I mean, quite a lot of the group wondered why I had reacted to her original compliment to the student in such a, in a feeling that I'd done something wrong.

Dr I.   You . . . . to recognise them.

Dr L.   Yes.

Dr O.   And you reacted this time to her wish for your immortality by saying 'What kind of a punishment is that?'

Dr L.   Exactly, exactly, yes.

Dr H.   That's the way you've been brought up in our groups, you can't take it all at its face-value any more.

E.B.   This is all what we've been doing to him over the last twenty years?

Dr H.   I'm afraid so. I think many of us thought that, you know, this was a genuine feeling of warmth, and that's the last thing we can accept, but anyway, she's come back with it, and even then you ungraciously acknowledge it. Next time around, perhaps you'll say/

Dr L.   I'll just enjoy it, you're saying?

Dr H.   No, you'll say 'thank you'/

Dr L.   OK Henry/

Dr H.   or not.

Dr L.   I may be still capable of learning, I'm not sure.

Dr O.   He may have taken an early retirement.

Dr J.   I still don't understand how did they get to you, both of them, on that morning? Because wasn't it just before they came to you, she had a little talk with Wayne? Or . . . .

Dr L.   Yes.

Dr J.   So how did she make the appointment? Or had she?

Dr L.   Well, she didn't make an appointment. She'd made an appointment for herself, that was, the appointment was for her.

Dr J.   Oh I see.

Dr L.   On Monday morning.

Dr J.   I'm with you.

Dr L.   And Wayne was not due, wasn't due in fact until an evening appointment next week, but because – she'd obviously had the talk and brought him along to her appointment.

Dr I.   Put him in the patient's chair.

Dr J.   Funny that she knew that you were worried about the two of them.

E.B.   Yes . . . . . I think so.

Dr L.   Sorry, I didn't hear what you said?

Dr J.   Funny that she knew you were worried about the two of them – to each other.

E.B.   She picked it up, yes, sure.

Dr O.   And even the way in which you were worried about them, the areas of worry came out, quite interesting.

E.B.   And you said like that 'Too hard on him' you know and you'd told us.

Dr L.   Yes.

E.B.   She picked that up and you must have conveyed it to her. We didn't know you had, I don't think we did, did we? We'll look at our script.

Dr O.   No.

Dr R.   She's a very perceptive woman, capable of making very personal remarks to her doctor. I mean she's obviously capable of talking straight to her son as well. But to go back to that remark, why did you feel that was such an odd thing to respond to it with?

Dr L.   You mean – with?

Dr R.   This latest one.

Dr H.   The response odd, or her comment?

Dr L.   Which response?

Dr O.   Yours.

Dr R.   Your response.

Dr L. About being chained?

Dr R. About the post.

Dr L. I don't know. It seemed a bit odd. I didn't know where it came from, really.

Dr H. Have you got an idea?

Dr R. Well, no I mean, it just didn't seem that odd to me, I mean it was about the retirement, wasn't it rather than the patient?

Dr L. Yes, yes.

Dr R. And previously, the problem had been with the patient, you couldn't take the patient's, personal problems.

Dr I. Who gets tied to the post, was the way you put it wasn't it?

Dr H. I mean, I would have said something about 'dying in harness' or . . . . but this is equivalent, isn't it?

Dr L. Mm, mm.

Dr I. Well tied to the post . . . . rather doglike.

E.B. She really values you.

Dr R. It confirms what we were thinking last time, that it, there was some genuine feeling, in the remark previously.

E.B. {Speaking as if she is the patient} 'Thank goodness you're not letting me think he's being awful. You realised that he's not being awful, I'm being awful.' She picked it all up, this girl.

Dr L. Mm, she was way ahead of me, obviously.

Dr H. Were you worried, or was it just some of us, about the aggressive relationship that she might have had with the son?

Dr L. The group were more worried than I was.

Dr H. Yes, but now we're saying that she's perceived your worry about it now. Were you wanting it both ways?

E.B. I was worried.

Dr L. No, no I'm not – I didn't think that she'd been physically violent, but I thought that she'd been very, you know, a martinet towards Wayne. Enid was worried she'd actually struck him, but in the circumstances, I couldn't possibly/

Dr J. Is it the surprise you had when you actually realised the boy was deaf, truly deaf?

Dr L. Yes.

Dr J. Made her felt as/

Dr L. Swine.

Dr H. Sorry, felt what?

Dr L. That she was horrible, because he was truly deaf.

Dr H. Yes, and know about the truth of that.

Dr J. She's been a bad mother.

Dr H. I mean you're not sure.

E.B.   Would she be able to take . . . . .

Dr L. Well, I think, he certainly is deaf but the interesting thing was that I had considered that he gave me very accurate answers the first time round.

Dr H. Did you record this apparent improvement in the tests?

Dr L. Yes.

Dr N. There's only one thing that troubles me, Leonard, about the story, and it hasn't got anything to do with the patient really; it's about this silent button. I'm so intrigued by the mechanics of 'the silent button'. That doesn't seem to – I mean, what does it do?

Dr H. High technology.

Dr L. Well, no it isn't, with the little audiogram, you know you press things, and you see they can visualise it, as it happens, when you're pressing.

Dr O. They can nod.

Dr L. There is in fact a button which gives a boost, so you could push an in-between button, because . . . . .

Dr N. So you can't – but they shouldn't be able to see you when you're doing it, should they?

Dr L. Well, they shouldn't, but in the . . . . it's not, it's not a very, I mean it's all done in the consulting room, it's nothing special about it. You should do it behind their back, but going down to the treatment room of a morning, is . . . . well, it wouldn't even be silent. It's better to do it where it is.

Dr N. I'm with you. I've got a picture of it now.

Dr O. It's a sort of placebo button, isn't it? You can press/

Dr L. Yes, if you only press the boost button actually no sound comes at all. But it looks as if you're doing the same thing.

Dr O. Yes. So if the patient nods, you know they're sprucing.

Dr L. Yes, that's right.

E.B.   I mean, do we want to find fault with his treatment, because I, it's a nonsense to find fault. It went terribly well, you know, you didn't have to give her a talk about her fears about being awful to . . . . this, her son and she's frightened she's damaged him or been too hard; because she did that without you and without any more help. You can't expect, I mean, you can't want anything better than that, I think that's absolutely marvellous.

Dr O. I think it's not a question of finding fault at all, I absolutely, but I'd like to be able to spell out more what you did that was right.

E.B.   Mm, mm.

Dr L. What I want to do is to make, if I get this thing, make a judgement of it, and not luck, if you see what I mean.

Dr O.   That's right, that's exactly what I mean, I don't think it was luck. I do believe it was judgement, but it's sharing it consciously with us.

Dr H.   I think it was an intuitive judgement and/

E.B.   What, Henry?

Dr H.   Intuitive judgement. I don't know what you think of this scenario, but I think you laid it on thick, on the basis of something, which on reflection was unclassifiable. One test on a home-made gadget and you let her have it; whether you let her have it, she took it, and full of remorse. Now I think that worked, the oracle, that was the very beginning of it; and whether or not you conspired, I still don't know, because now you see, you haven't got the force of that test, and whether she will feel something towards you – 'Well you told me last time that he was very deaf and now, you know'. Has she talked about it? No.

Dr L.   I didn't say he was very deaf, I said he was definitely deaf, and I said this time that he was better, and I said, 'And it's only three weeks and not four weeks'.

Dr H.   Quite . . . . Well, it worked.

E.B.   I think what was all right about it was that she was reprimanded not by your having said anything but just by your saying he was deaf; but you still went on liking her; I mean, she can't have felt you thought 'My God, what a frightful woman, I'd better give her a good talking to'. She must have felt that you were still with her, otherwise she wouldn't have made that remark about what a splendid doctor you were. You did something to make her feel liked, despite the fact that she'd been awful, which we're always trying to do with our patients.

Dr N.   I mean I felt that was the bit – I don't think that was intuition. I think that was conscious skill, and the thought that she made that remark and you, it was just so. It just fitted what you felt about it. It was hearing what she had to say, but it wasn't actually interpreting it as if she was making a conscious attack on you. It actually, it sprang from her and you treated it appropriately.

E.B.   Leonard didn't have to do anything except say the boy was deaf. I mean, he wasn't being terribly skilful in saying this, 'You know you're to blame' or anything of that kind, he just had to say he was deaf, but not look as if he was horrified at what she was doing – which he wasn't. I believe when we talk about being frightened of saying something quite casual, it is because we are shocked at the idea of . . . . I mean you can't say something if it shocks you when you say it.

Dr O.   Something about, the intimacy of what you're saying and getting in too close; some of the things that Enid's been talking about that she is braver at saying – certainly than I would be – has to do with, I think, daring to be that intimate.

E.B.   Well taking it for granted that people are whatever it is.

Dr O.   Yes.

Dr N.   That's right . . . .

E.B.   It does require a kind of intimacy it's true, but it's/

Dr L.   It's got to be within the context of a very free and open relationship, that like friends who can say things. I mean, a friend who can't tell you bad news is no friend, that kind of . . . .

Dr H.   Yes.

Dr O.   Yes.

Dr H.   Funnily enough, I saw it not as an expression of intimacy, but of the distance, which allows you this room. Whereas utter closeness, I don't think could do.

Dr L.   Is it a balance? That I've, it's a professional statement – 'Wayne is deaf to a certain extent. On the other hand I'm not casting you out because you thought he was sprucing.'

Dr H.   If you were that close, you would begin to wonder 'Now what would a statement of deafness mean to this poor woman? . . . . No I can't inflict this on her.' You know.

Dr O.   Yes, that's my point.

E.B.   I must protect her from this ghastly news.

Dr H.   Yes, but he was being thoroughly professional. Maybe he was calling a spade a spade/

E.B.   You see, it's a very good example of what we're trying to do and we can have it without making Leonard feel embarrassed because really you didn't have to do anything carefully at all.

Dr L.   Blundered about like an elephant.

E.B.   You actually didn't blunder about, but it wasn't a long skilful tortuous affair.

Dr N.   Isn't the thing which actually stops us being – stops us blundering about – is if when we come up with words that we want to use which are slightly judgemental, so I mean, you could say to her for example, 'Yes, he's deaf' – without thinking of the implication of the judgement – 'It's you that's caused it by batting him round the ear' or whatever it is. And as soon as we get into a framework within ourselves and pondering it and thinking about it and coming up with judgemental words, it's then that we don't have the courage to, say it because/

Dr L.   Yes, because the exchange could be said – Mother brings child saying, 'He says he's deaf', all right? Doctor tests. Responds, 'Yes!

he is deaf.' Mother responds, 'My God! I didn't think he was deaf. What have I done? Isn't the doctor marvellous.' Doctor responds, 'My God, what an awful mess *I* have made' – in that sense, so invites mother to come back, in her own right in order to try and clear it up.

Dr N.   Right.

Dr H.   I'd like to/

E.B.   Mother did decide that in order not to get a dressing down she'd have it out with her son first, which is very good but, it was in order not to be/

Dr O.   It's very interesting because one of the options was – was there to be a joint interview, and they had one. [Laughter]

Dr L.   I didn't arrange it.

Dr O.   That's right.

Dr L.   They arranged it, yes.

Dr H.   I'd like to suggest that this could give us a focus for our studies or research. That instead of, because it was thought last time or the time before, that it might help to modify our techniques. Now instead of teaching each other to suck eggs – grandmothers or not – why don't we employ what's so obviously manifest, that somehow we *know*, but what we don't know is *how* we know; and if we could explore the intimacies of this case, we would learn a lot more about how we sometimes, unerringly, seem to be on the right track, or choose an option. Not 'You should change, you should do something or other', as we've been saying to Ian {Referring back to the case that has just been presented by Ian and discussed in the first part of this meeting} but what it is about the case and his handling, that seems to be appropriate for that situation. So in other words, instead of the reformists' zeal, I think we should be there as learners, although I know Ian felt criticised, we were struggling to understand what was going on. That should be a focus, I think, for our group, because there's a lot we don't understand.

Dr L.   Of our apparently automatic responses.

Dr H.   That's right. The things we're ashamed of.

Dr O.   Which may be better than we know.

Dr H.   The soft data, the shameful hunches.

E.B.   I think we do know, actually . . . . . . I think, you didn't have to think this out, but you knew you didn't want to make this woman feel awful that her son was deaf. I think we do usually know; there's no earthly point in making patients feel awful. I mean we, I think this was kind of chapter one of the first book but it was made in terms of apostolic functions and judgements, and now we're talking about it in terms of taking it for granted that there's no point in making patients feel awful about what they've done. Can't we take that as read, really? We know that.

Dr H.   No, you see, Leonard said that he'd just blundered into this happy situation. Well, I don't think he blundered. There is no evidence of it.

E.B.   No, I don't think it's a blunder. The actual words to you he said were, but they come up, well blunders if you like; he didn't make up his mind he was going to say that, but if we make up our minds what we're going to say it comes out flat as a pancake anyway.

Dr O.   That's right.

E.B.   It's got to be spontaneous and it can only be spontaneous because we know inside ourselves what we want to convey.

Dr L.   Mm, mm.

Dr O.   And it feels right at that moment.

Dr L.   Yes . . . .

E.B.   And why is it so difficult to know? . . . . . Terribly simple, isn't it?

Dr L.   The trouble is perhaps it is because of this damn, I mean, although Henry cursed Janet for not being professional {Referring to yet another case, this time presented by Janet}, perhaps in fact there is a great danger, because then if you have to consider everything and put it into professional-ese, that will lose the spontaneity; you have to react as the doctor-person you are.

E.B.   But you've got to be the right kind of doctor-person, 'Yes, oh I'll be judgemental' like that.

Dr L.   True.

E.B.   I mean, if you are a judgemental type doctor, well you are. You'll act on it. There is no point in not acting on it, because it won't/

Dr H.   Yes, I agree. But I don't think Leonard is programmed to be exactly the same with every patient, or with the same patient every time, and I think he laced that, I think he laced that judgement about the deafness, and we don't know because we weren't there, but I suspect it was, just that – with just a tint of acerbity. I'm not sure?

Dr L.   I have a feeling you're right, yes.

Dr H.   You certainly didn't do it with a smile 'Oh, that's all right, he's definitely deaf'.

Dr L.   Yes, I was protecting Wayne, that is . . . that is an emotion I remember. So you're/

Dr H.   And it worked, absolutely.

E.B.   But she brought him so that, I mean, that was her plan – set it up that way. OK well thank you very much.

{Discussion about this case finished here}

Report of first follow-up

Leonard gave a follow-up on Angela Denton. She returned (to his surprise) with a cheerful looking Wayne. A hearing test revealed improvement. She apologised for her behaviour at the last consultation, attributing it to 'PMT'. She had been able to have a lengthy discussion with her son, resulting in an improved relationship. Leonard, on questioning Wayne, felt this was genuine. On leaving, she remarked, 'You must never retire!' Leonard replied, 'You want me to be chained to the post for ever!' [Written by Dr H.]

Points emerging from the discussion

1 Last week Leonard had been sceptical about an apparent compliment; he responded rather ungraciously to the present one
2 In the first consultation he had successfully conveyed, and she had accurately detected, his anxiety about the aggressive quality in the mother–son relationship.
3 She felt reprimanded by Leonard, but knew also that she was still liked by him.
4 He had achieved a great deal. Whether intuitively or by blundering (Leonard's term) it reflected experience, professional concern for both of his patients and a feeling for them as human beings.
5 Was there any need to quibble with Leonard's technique?

SECTION C

Second follow-up: Seminar No.16 (25.4.85)

E.B.   Well, let's have a follow-up.

Dr L.   I've got a follow-up, but has anybody else, I mean/

E.B.   We've got/

Dr L.   If somebody has got a new one?

E.B.   No one?

Dr N.   I had a, well no perhaps I/

E.B.   Shall we have a couple of follow-ups, we will start with Leonard.

Dr L.   Right, well this is a follow-up on Wayne Denton. You remember with the mother who, the student and the ears and the arguments and everything. You remember the thing that was left as it were on, on the map, was that he was coming back to have his ears tested. Do you remember?

E.B.   Um, yes.

Dr L.   He duly appeared with mum to have his ears tested and I duly tested the ears and I considered his hearing was back to normal and this is the sort of, and then as, when I sort of said, 'I think his hearing is fine', Angela said to me, 'But now there is something else that he's been complaining of being out of breath when he plays sport. And I've said to him don't be silly you know you are inventing something else.' She actually said this you see, so I looked at Wayne who actually smiled, because it is now in the open, if you see what I mean, the, and in some way, I said, 'Look, tell me what it is about?' . . . . and it is quite clear that whenever he exercises he gets breathless and so I have a nice little toy which I call the elephant. It's the Vitalograph, and he clearly has exercise asthma, because I got him to double up and down the treatment room and blow in the machine and so on and it is also reversible with Intal, cromoglycate. And he came back, I had instructed him on what to do; and he came back a week later and he said he had been markedly better but he did not like the taste of cromoglycate, which is actually disgusting and lots of children don't like it. So in fact I gave him a corticosteroid inhaler instead, and that . . . um . . . worked perfectly alright and he complies with it, he does not mind taking it. He takes, he takes a dose before his break, when he has to charge about and another dose after lunch before he has his afternoon sort of games and things. But it was, as far as I was concerned, it is just simple maintenance as far as I can see; but the interesting thing was that this thing which had been going on at least until the beginning of the academic year, last

	year in September, when he went to his new secondary school had not brought to the doctor's attention until this particular interview.
E.B.	Um.
Dr H.	How old is he?
Dr L.	He is eleven plus, he is coming up to twelve. [7 seconds silence]
E.B.	Has he been hanging on to it or has his mother?
Dr L.	That is a good question. I think that he had said it to his mother. I am sure this is true but because she had not been listening to what, any of his complaints very much. It had got, he had not actually pressed it but I think that was the nearest point.
E.B.	Um.
Dr L.	The interesting thing is his exercise-induced asthma certainly does not seem to be relieved by the new mother–child relationship shift. I mean it isn't better, but I don't think it is particularly . . . . .
Dr R.	But the other things happened.
Dr L.	Yes.
Dr R.	It had been allowed to emerge.
Dr L.	Yes.
Dr R.	And been treated. Surely that is the important/
Dr L.	I think that is the point, everything can now be/
Dr R.	Yes.
E.B.	That's very good.
Dr L.	One change has led to a free/
Dr R.	Presentation/
Dr L.	Presentation of another condition. [Dr R.: Yes.] Yes.
E.B.	It must mean the situation has changed in the relationship between the boy and his mother?
Dr L.	Yes.
Dr R.	Um.
E.B.	I would have thought, outside the surgery, the boy could show the mother. The mother could see and this must, I would say it must, but I would have thought must reflect in their relationship generally. Wouldn't that be what we would expect?
Dr L.	That would certainly be what I would have observed. I mean they are quite different. They were quite, quite different in the, in that consultation about, when they had brought back for the hearing, than they had been before. There was an openness, the lack of hostility and sort of tension on both sides, is . . . . you can feel it.
E.B.	Look, can I just say one thing as I think it is relevant to our research, which is that in some groups, in groups of psychiatrists and also psychotherapist groups, and also in some GP groups, once the word asthma is mentioned everybody kind of says, good, good now we

know that he is angry and hostile and one would begin, you know, because asthma is meant to be a symptom of hostility and anger, and immediately that would be what was being discussed; *not* changes due to what has been going on and the relationship between the mother and child. In other words the boy is freer. It is a difference but it's not that we ignore the other, but we are not talking about it . . . . .

Dr L.   We know he has been angry with his mother on the one hand and it would fit in but it also can . . . . . . but angry feelings can be now aired.

E.B.   It will be interesting how long the asthma lasts.

Dr H.   He has had it six months you said?

Dr L.   Yes, the thing, that of course, he may have had it much longer on the basis that at secondary school they take much more exercise at school. I mean formal exercise, than they do at primary schools in my neck of the woods, and therefore it has only been a problem to him since he went to secondary school.

E.B.   Wouldn't asthma show without exercise?

Dr L.   Exercise? This is a particular subgroup of asthma which seems to. I mean it is, so far, in his case it is. Only when he exercises does he get the wheeze.

Dr H.   Well, it has got to start sometime.

Dr L.   Absolutely.

Dr H.   And it has got to be reported sometime.

Dr L.   Um.

Dr H.   I am not sure if I can go along with – 'allow the case to be brought up' – unless you are using the word allow in some way that I don't understand. There may have been some discretion on the mother's part, one thing at a time.

Dr L.   True.

Dr H.   Certainly if I had been overloaded with a dozen symptoms, I would have said first things first. Just get the [Mumble] then tell me about this when you come in.

Dr N.   Could we just go back? When you reported it I was so overcome with the sense of disbelief, my observatory powers were suspended when you were telling [Dr L.: Yes] what actually . . . . I mean, I sensed that it happened to you too, about yet another physical thing and a sense of disbelief.

Dr L.   Yes.

Dr N.   Could you just tell me? I wasn't listening properly [Dr L.: Um.] to what you had to say. How did, I mean you laughed with them about it did you? You sort of/

Dr L.   I tested his ears, that's what the contract was. Okay, and then, and then his, Angela said, 'There is something else that he has told me. I'd like you to, I would like your opinion on' or something of that sort and 'that is that he says that he gets very uncomfortable when he plays games at school'.

Dr N.   Um.

E.B.   Instead of saying there, there.

Dr L.   Yes, yes and so, I looked at Wayne and he was sort of quite relaxed and smiling at this point, and then I asked him to tell me about what happened.

Dr H.   You did not announce your scepticism? This is what Nick was asking.

Dr L.   No.

Dr H.   No, I see.

Dr L.   But no!

Dr N.   No, I didn't. I think it wasn't the scepticism about whether he had the breathlessness. It was whether he . . . . 'Oh! here we go again'. It was a sort of sense of déjà vu.

Dr L.   Oh! I see/

Dr N.   Of/

Dr L.   Yes/

Dr N.   Of, er/

Dr L.   I'm with you/

Dr N.   With her saying he says he/

Dr L.   You think, 'Oh my God! here we go again'.

Dr N.   *He* says he is short of breath/

Dr L.   I remained supremely optimistic throughout [Dr N.: Yes] don't, I didn't, I am not sure I can explain, I take your point, you just think Oh! God! here we go again.

Dr H.   Well you said that. What did you mean by what you said? You joked and laughed about it but [Dr L.: Yes] was that just to yourself or to her? That is what Nick and I are asking.

Dr L.   Oh! I see.

E.B.   I took it that he read, that, took it all differently. I took it and Leonard thought, well certainly there is something wrong, [Dr L.: Yes] and I will examine it . . .

Dr L.   Yes, that was my view.

E.B.   With the boy.

Dr H.   It was your experience with her?

E.B.   Because of the ears.

Dr L.   Yes, yes.

Dr N.   I mean, I took it that was so.

Dr L.   Yes.

Dr N.   But there was a sort of, a sense of in me of where you were before when she had come about the hearing [Dr L.: I see] and said he says he cannot hear.

Dr L.   No, no I wasn't. I didn't feel, you remember I put my foot in it. I felt there was something that, when she alerted me, I didn't feel that, that . . . . . . those reservations that I had in the first time. I had a feeling that the communication between Wayne and Angela was on a different level now.

Dr N.   Yes, I thought that the different level was a tacit assumption between you. Oh! here we are again but we can go on and take it seriously and that's it.

Dr R.   I don't think that. I think the difference in level of communication was that the parent and child were much more open and similarly you, in the consulting room, were much open to take it at face-value.

Dr L.   Yes, that's absolutely, that is how I see it. [Dr R.: Um] There wasn't any playing games, or is he really deaf, or is he not listening. There was nothing of that I took/

Dr N.   But when you told him with a sense of fun.

Dr H.   Yes, you said.

Dr L.   Did I?

Dr H.   There is nothing the matter with him, what was that about?

Dr L.   Nothing the matter with him?

Dr H.   Yes.

Dr R.   No he didn't.

Dr N.   No.

Dr L.   I never said that.

Dr H.   When you looked at him and laughed?

Dr L.   No, no!

E.B.   On the contrary.

Dr L.   *He* laughed, I looked at him and *he* laughed. He smiled at me, he was a different boy. He was a sullen boy the first time he came in.

Dr N.   Ah! The sense of fun was in him?

Dr L.   The sense of fun was in him not in me.

Dr N.   Right.

Dr L.   Yes.

Dr G.   I don't think it is, well what do you mean by face-value? Do you mean perhaps it is a physical, you know, true physical symptom, reflecting physical illness? Because I mean the way I see it is that the relationship between the boy and the mother has changed, so that whether or not it reflected a true physical illness or it was psychological, the mother and the boy could both deal with either of these outcomes. [Dr L.: Um]

E.B. Yes.

Dr G. It wouldn't matter which.

Dr L. It was entirely free of what it was, yes, I/

Dr R. That's what I meant by face-value, yes.

E.B. This is the perfect case isn't it? One for our research, can be physical or needn't be and . . .

Dr L. Um.

Dr G. And you can still/

E.B. I mean there it is.

Dr H. It is also the perfect case for what Ruth wanted, because we have had five different versions of what it means. So that what's actually said. [Laughter and yes's from several which drown Henry for 10 seconds] No, really.

E.B. Are they all different really?

Dr L. Yes, they are, actually, yes. It is true. Well, no. Some group themselves. I mean Henry and Nick were, are quite, and you and Ruth, and Gaby and I'm not quite sure which subgroup/

Dr N. [Laughs] Yes, I know, you were trying to lump me with Henry.

Dr L. [Laughs] then others/

Dr H. Seriously, I don't know, what to think really about it, but I am/

E.B. You must/

Dr H. /sceptical about it.

E.B. This is very important because I don't see this and you do which is, this is something that I don't observe.

Dr H. I mean, you were very quick to grasp that this is evidence of a, the relationship, not between the doctor and the patient which is interesting, but between, you know this is the third party again, those two are getting on so well together, that it has allowed something to be brought up, which by inference, would not have been.

Dr L. But it is more than that. It is not just the patient and the mother, it is me as well. We were all absolutely in the ring together [Dr N.: Um] completely relaxed. That's the feeling.

Dr H. So the mother sensed that you were accessible.

Dr L. Yes, but and not, not . . . . . you remember, I took her remark to the student, rightly or wrongly, but I took, as a question I'd somehow left her out of the original consultation and had been really on the side of Wayne against her. This time it was absolutely equal and that is to say that nobody had any sort of hidden agenda in what was being said. It was that, it was the absolutely fascinating thing to me then that I, and I didn't get the feeling of Oh, God! here we go again, or anything like. I didn't have any negative feeling at all. I was just, I thought this is something, you know we are all agreeing that this must be examined.

Dr H.   So it didn't need a mallet to draw your attention to something. But I can't see you as ever requiring a mallet.

Dr L.   Very kind.

Dr R.   But hadn't the mallet been applied before?

Dr H.   Well, had it?

Dr R.   Perhaps the student, I mean who knows what the mallet was. We are not quite sure but it happened before [Mumbled].

Dr H.   Something was reported on this occasion, which could have been, which was not reported earlier. Now it seems to me that Leonard is making a lot out of that, er it may be true, but is [Mumbled].

Dr L.   Exactly, I take your point.

Dr H.   I want to know how you can justify? I mean, I believe it, but er is it a matter of belief only or can we say 'Look, *how* do we know?'

Dr L.   He had clearly complained to his mother before I, before the very first consultation about the difficulty. She had dismissed that like his deafness, I think. I am looking at that retrospectively you understand, but my feeling was that he's been complaining of, about this since last September, so that was a long time before.

Dr H.   She has taken him seriously.

Dr L.   Yes.

Dr H.   Now.

Dr L.   Yes.

Dr H.   So I think your therapy really has been on the mother.

Dr L.   Yes, yes . . . . . I would go along with that . . . . . .

Dr R.   Do you think there is a way that we can ask patients to establish whether the changes that we see are/

Dr H.   Well, I don't/

Dr R.   real changes?

Dr H.   No, it's by repeated observation, this is the main strength of our work, the follow-ups.

Dr R.   Um.

Dr H.   Going to months and sometimes years which we must never underestimate.

Dr R.   Yes, but the change we are looking at here is whether there was asthma for a long time and mother was just ignoring this even though the boy was mentioning it? That's the information that would help us determine whether a real change had occurred.

Dr H.   You see what worries me is I have got patients where there is no capacity for absorbing anything, so as soon as a child transmits to the mother it is reflected straight to me. There is no way in which it's considered or let's see how you get on. You know the sort of thing I mean.

Dr L. Mm.

Dr H. I don't know whether her behaviour is of a good mother containing it, until it becomes a matter of prudence to do something else or not.

Dr L. Yes.

Dr H. So how? What can you do Leonard to/

Dr L. [Sighs] Yes/

Dr H. elicit the barrier, shall we say if it is a barrier, to her revealing to you earlier on? Was it her preoccupation with the other thing, the ear trouble? Which for her may be a much more grisly spectre than exertional dyspnoea.

E.B. Well, I would have thought it was something. An upside down of what it used to be. The mother thought this was a load of neurotic rubbish [Dr L.: Um] and so said to the boy, 'Don't be absurd, you are perfectly alright'. Whereas before we used to see cases where the mother thought it was a serious physical condition and the doctor said it was a lot of rubbish. [Dr L. chuckles] This case is . . . um . . . alright. We take this seriously. I feel that the strange thing about it is that, having got as far as that, there are lots of questions in my mind. I would like now to *know* about the mother's relationship with the child. What is going on? And also, is the child playing the mother up? And you know lots of other questions, but we, being GPs, can wait to find out. But these must be questions, if we report this, everybody wants to know. 'Why didn't you find out? What's been happening between the mother and the child?' and 'Is he being very hostile to her?' and er, . . . but we are only interested in, at the moment, in examining and looking and observing the changes in the boy with his mother in relation to his physical symptoms, and that is all we are looking at. We're excluding all else. It is fair enough.

Dr L. Um.

Dr H. Well, Leonard has testified that he himself has changed and he observes change in each of the two and in their relationship, so um, we've got three people here who have changed, manifestly.

Dr L. What Enid said, I mean, is certainly relevant because when I thought of doing the follow-up, you know, ... but this is real general practice. When I'd done the spirometry thing, and I felt I had done enough and when he comes back and it's working that is not enough and that, of course, is only symptom control and that is all I am doing. [E.B.: Yes.] And there is no doubt that I am, you might say, that I was also aware that there may be a can of worms, the lid of which I did not wish to take off at the moment, thank you very much. But there it is.

E.B.   Yes, it was appropriate, because of the previous interchange, just to deal with that symptom.

Dr L.   Yes.

Dr R.   But is it appropriate or a selective neglect?

Dr L.   Well selective neglect, yes. Well, it could be both of course.

E.B.   But it wasn't unconscious.

Dr L.   I mean it could be appropriate selective neglect. It was conscious.

E.B.   It was consciously selective neglect [Dr L.: Yes] very different from unconscious.

Dr G.   The same thing, you could say about the hearing because you could have said, 'This hearing is now normal, do you think he hears you any better?' [Dr L.: Oh, yes!] I mean, you actually . . . . . it's all that area.

E.B.   Fascinating.

Dr L.   Yes, absolutely, yes.

Dr N.   What about medication, I was just interested in your choice, a few points and/

E.B.   Yes, do tell me about it.

Dr L.   Is it?

Dr N.   No, I just, are there other choices that you could have made?

Dr L.   Well, pre-pubertal children I usually start with cromoglycate, er . . . [Dr N.: Right, fine] and then I proceed to Becotide.

Dr N.   You don't like Ventolin.

E.B.   What would you have done?

Dr N.   I mean, I just wondered if salbutamol

Dr L.   Would have been enough?

Dr N.   Which is the same as Ventolin [Dr L.: Yes] I mean, I just wondered whether you, whether that was your standard practice or whether/

Dr L.   My standard practice with exercise-induced [Dr H.: Explain to the] because I want to, yes. The thing is that, there is the one that just reverses the airway [E.B.: Um] spasm, which is that, which is what Nick said, 'Why didn't I use?' It's a good question. My own feeling is that I want to, for longer cover, I tend to/

Dr H.   This, sodium cromoglycate [Dr L.: Maybe] for allergic asthma, that it was then found to be useful for exercise-induced asthma, against all the predictions.

Dr L.   Yes.

E.B.   What is? I mean, what side effects do you have?

Dr L.   None at all.

Dr H.   No, it either works or it doesn't.

Dr N.   And what, in which way did you give, did you give it as a rotacap or a spray?

Dr L.   The Becotide? [Dr N.: Um] I gave it as a rotacap, but that was more because I'd given him the Intal, but I thought it might be easier to explain rather than/

E.B.   Is it one of those syringe things?

Dr L.   No it is just a sort of inhaler. You, you suck it in.

Dr H.   It's not out of pressure. Yes, it is easily controlled.

Dr N.   I think it is actually quite a complicated routine [Dr L.: Yes] for a kid to get hold of. You have to spend quite a lot of time actually talking to them about it. It isn't exactly quite the same as Intal, er I mean you have to explain how to use the machine.

E.B.   Well, I have got a thirty-five-year-old man who is addicted to his. You can imagine.

Dr H.   This is why I think if Leonard/

E.B.   This is why I was asking what side effects.

Dr H.   Yes, what Intal, Oh! Ventolin. I have gone off Ventolin, I must say, but you know this is going to be three or four times a day, er, irrespective of symptoms [Dr L.: Three times a day, yes] so rather than something you take when you feel you need it [Dr L.: Yes] you have got to take it before you need it [Dr L.: Yes] which again fits the different/

Dr L.   Yes.

E.B.   It must be better otherwise you are always reaching out for it.

Dr H.   So a bit of health education is necessary, you have to talk to really, literally talk them into doing it.

Dr L.   You do, yes and he didn't and because the Intal tastes nasty, he gave it up in spite of the fact that it did good.

Dr H.   There are two Intals as you know and there is the one/

Dr L.   plain . . . .

E.B.   We have concentrated, not now, just the one relationship aspect of it. There are heaps of other things because what does it mean to the mother having not a deaf child but an asthmatic? [Laughter] So really I thought that a woman having a deaf child which she hasn't and . . . .

Dr H.   That's interesting. This, because we haven't enquired what her reaction was, to the implications [E.B.: No] has she asked you, 'Will this go on forever doctor? Will he grow out of it?'

E.B.   No.

Dr L.   About the deafness or the asthma?

Dr H.   No, the asthma. Did you mention the dread word [Dr L.: Yes] or did you say as I might have done, 'wheezy bronchitis'?

Dr L.   No, I have sort of got a thing about saying, calling asthma, asthma.

Dr H.   So what did she say? How did she respond to that?

E.B.　[Mumbles]

Dr H.　Well, it must be from the father's side!

Dr L.　Yes! [Roars of laughter] How did you guess?

Dr H.　We are understanding this woman I think, [More laughter and bit mumbled] which is another facet of our group work. I'd be quite interested, how we so closely identify and can recognise those patients as if they were our own and indeed they are . . . .

Dr L.　Yes, I had forgotten that. I asked her, 'Not in my family', says Mrs Denton [More laughter] . . . . But I can justifiably say that it is extremely mild and some people only wheezed when they did take exercise.

E.B.　And I think you will have to remember to tell me all this kind of thing because this I don't know about. I might have come across it but . . .

Dr L.　Fair enough, yes. [10 seconds silence]

E.B.　Well, thank you that's, we have got a quarter of an hour, anybody got a brief one?

{Discussion on Mrs Denton and Wayne finished here}

Report of second follow-up

Wayne returned with his mother for a hearing test, which proved normal. Mother reported that for about six months Wayne had been getting out of breath when playing sports. He actually looked well and was smiling, but Leonard was alerted and was able to demonstrate the presence of exercise-induced asthma reversible with Intal rotacaps. Because Wayne disliked the taste of the latter, a steroid inhaler was substituted later. [Written by Dr H.]

Discussion

1　Was news of the breathing difficulty held back because of mother's scepticism? consideration of the doctor? or preoccupation with Wayne's hearing problem?

2　Or had the strikingly changed mother–child relationship, with its absence of tension and hostility, now 'allowed' the reporting of Wayne's asthma?

3　Evidently the improved relationship had not helped the asthma.

4　What about the impact on the mother of the diagnosis? It was predicted she would disclaim responsibility, and Leonard confirmed this: 'Not from my side of the family!'

SECTION D

Report of third follow-up: Seminar No.43 (30.1.86)

Wayne was brought for another hearing test (normal). Leonard asked about the asthma, mother answered that she had bought a book on food allergies, and he had been clear of asthma since avoiding yellow chicken. Wayne looked glum. Leonard winked at him and asked if it was too awful being off chicken. He then agreed that the chest was better and finished with, 'If things change come and see me.' [Written by Dr R.]

Discussion

1 Did Leonard undermine her by siding with Wayne, and was this a pattern from earlier consultations?
2 Leonard was nettled that she was being a better doctor than him, and had come to tell him how well he was doing
3 Who is the patient? Should Leonard concentrate on the mother–child relationship as the patient?
4 There seemed to be some competitiveness between Leonard and Mum, was he to be thrown out soon? This reminded Leonard that she now had a steady boyfriend.

Discussion of third follow-up report: Seminar No.44 (6.2.86)

[The beginning of the discussion had been about whether or not we have a technique with our patients.]

E.B. . . . . we have been discussing techniques all the time; skills. Skills is just as good a word.

Dr H. Yes. If we take Leonard's follow-up, with that thing that we seized on – his winking – and identifying that child as the one who is going to absorb my interest. Now, then we put forward an alternative, the gap between the doctor, er the mother and the child should be [the focus]. Now would you call these different techniques? Your winking is it a technique?

Dr L. Well, it's a . . . it is a technique, but unfortunately it came just, as you said, from parts of me that I am only dimly aware of. [Dr N.: Right] Having said that, that is what I did and I have done the same sort of thing twice. So this pair, the mother and the child, or the triangle somehow puts pressure on me to [Dr N.: Right] behave in a particular way. The thing is whether that is the best way to help everybody concerned and I/

E.B.   Are your skills very good? Is it a good skill or a bad skill? [Dr L.: Absolutely] What is a good skill, is looking at it. [Dr L.: Yes] The whole, what we are here for is not whether we did that well or badly [Dr L.: Quite] but to look at that as a skill; to be able to examine oneself, whether one did well that time or not, or whether one's in some kind of groove which one can't get out of. [Dr L.: Yes] That is most definitely a skill.

Dr G.   Is one of the problems with the word that technique sounds conscious? [E.B.: Mm] Well prejudged [Others make noises of agreement and Dr L.: I think that's possible] like 'Shall I wink at that child?' and then winked.

Dr H.   Definable.

Dr L.   It's a bit too cerebral?

Dr B.   It's overtone of trickery?

Dr L.   In fact Dan/

Dr B.   I don't think that this has it but it may be the thing that puts/

Dr H.   It means a well defined. I prefer what we've just heard, which is we are talking about observable behaviour. That's fine. If that's what technique means, then I will accept it.

E.B.   That is one of the ones; one of the techniques – to be able to examine what one's done and whether what one's done is right.

Dr H.   Yes, what one did.

E.B.   That's the basic technique I should say, but we've got masses of others.

Dr H.   Well, the reason that I'm seizing on this is that you only know in retrospect. Nick would not have predicted that his technique with that patient would be such and such; and Leonard would not say, 'Now tomorrow when he comes in I am going to wink at him'. Now that, a technique you can predict, that's why it's really/

Dr L.   But taking your point that, I quite accept what you've just said, the next time those two come I shall, I intend to be aware of trying to do something different. [Dr H.: Right] That is to say not identifying with the child against the mother. So I shall actually sort of, I'll probably fail, but I shall attempt to/

Dr H.   You know better than us that predictions used to be a feature of those forms [Dr L.: Yes] so let us predict our techniques, I don't think/

Dr I.   Actually I see winking, whether it was subconscious or conscious, was a technique. Understanding why he winked and what it meant/

E.B.   That is what I mean by technique [Dr L.: Yes] absolutely.

Dr H.   So you mean behaviour.

E.B.   No! It's not behaviour Henry. It isn't.

Dr L.   The idea underlying the behaviour. What I was trying to do.

Dr H.   So you can have unconscious techniques?

Dr L.   Yes, it's like driving you don't, you don't, or breathing.

Dr N.   Sorry, can I just follow it a little further, Henry? Technique as I see it, the technique that we have in this group, is to examine the behaviour [Dr H.: Yes] that was observed and is reported. Now part of the technique of that examination is to facilitate the reporter to describe what happened fully. Now if you can't facilitate that, you can't look at it, then this group doesn't have a technique.

E.B.   Not only observe the behaviour but the feelings that go with it [Dr N.: Yes] very important. Sorry to take up the group's time with this but I've just been puzzling about it and thought I'd better not stay awake at night any longer. Could we go on to something else? We can come back to this and no doubt we will, but what did we feel about Ruth's write up? Any comments?

{No more were offered and discussion about Mrs Denton and Wayne finished here at this meeting}

SECTION E

Report of fourth follow-up: Seminar No.53 (8.5.86)

They had come together again. Mrs Denton looking more made-up and Wayne slightly more cheerful. 'I'm afraid his allergies are all back.' Leonard saw a rather indeterminate rash and wasn't convinced that it was due to a true allergy, going on to enquire of Mrs Denton how her diet treatment was getting on. Wayne mentioned still not being allowed chicken legs and Mrs D. mentioned he also has pains, mainly in his elbows and knees. Wayne's joints were not painful when Leonard examined them and she said, 'I tell him they are growing pains'. This was a crunch dilemma for Leonard who normally does not allow the existence of growing pains but did not want to be yet again in the role of contradicting Mrs D. 'Maybe you're right' he managed and then arranged for them to be able to come back if Wayne's pains did not settle. [Written by Dr B.]

Discussion

1 Growing pains/growing-up pains/strains between Wayne and his mother.
2 Leonard was unable to explore this much and kept with the symptoms. He still feels over-identified with Wayne.
3 Who was the patient on this occasion?
4 Can Leonard open it up with these two more?
5 He would like to be able to see Mrs D. on her own. Perhaps she will arrange this as she did before.
6 Where is Wayne's father? Is he missing him and Mrs D. can't bear this so she is keeping the doctor out in the same way as she does Wayne's father?
7 It is a very delicately balanced relationship.

Discussion of fourth follow-up report: Seminar No.54 (15.5.86)

The seminar had opened with a discussion about research in general. Dr O. had not been there the previous week and was critical that there did not seem to be much of a research focus in the report of Seminar No.53. This was partly accepted; those at the previous meeting defended themselves; they had been looking at connections (a previously declared aim) or 'what went with what', both in the patient and between the patient and the doctor. The discussion had been going for about fifteen minutes when this was said:

E.B.   There was something also about Leonard's case I can't remember what it was . . . [Papers rustle] 'What went with what' was very unclear, but we wanted to know, in relation to Mrs Denton's relation to men and her relation to Wayne. There clearly are patterns but we don't know what they are.

Dr L.   All useful work by me was completely thrown out of the window at the cost of me stamping on identifying with Wayne against Mrs D. [E.B.: Yes] I mean because I, . . . having, . . . swallowing my feelings about 'growing pains', I completely blew everything else [Dr N.: And yet/] I didn't ask what she meant by 'growing pains'/

Dr N.   And yet when you identified with Wayne before, then the work moved forward.

Dr L.   Exactly, so I did the wrong thing.

E.B.   Yes [Dr N. chuckles].

Dr L.   I think I did the wrong thing.

E.B.   Yes, he did the wrong thing actually. I mean we've got to be able to say this, haven't we? Otherwise we are sunk.

Dr L.   I was terribly proud of myself for stamping on it. [Chuckles all round] Actually it was the wrong thing to do. [More chuckling] I should have said 'Growing pains!' [Loud laugh from Dr N. and chuckles from Dr L.]

{The group then went on to discuss the other cases in the report of Seminar No.53}

Report of discussion of fourth follow-up

Leonard had been proud of not stamping on Mrs Denton's 'growing-pains' concept, but had come to see it was a pity he had not stamped on it because that might have carried the work forward. Perhaps the doctor must be himself at all costs, and work from there? [Written by Dr L.]

SECTION F

Report of fifth follow-up: Seminar No.61 (25.9.86)

Seen routinely for oral contraception check. She reported no family disturbance. Her new boyfriend seems to be accepted by the boys (even Wayne). Wayne is well (the pains he complained of at the last contact went quickly). [Written by Dr L.]

Discussion

It seems she got permission to have a stable sexual relationship again. There is a man in the house again and she does not feel the need to be both parents any more.

SECTION G

Report of sixth follow-up: Seminar No.69 (11.12.86)

Mrs D. had said that Leonard had asked to see Wayne again. Leonard does not recall this. She has relaxed his exclusion diet, his hearing seems normal, his asthma under control and growing pains gone. She then sent him out of the room. She wanted a pill check, and said she was getting married next year. The only problem with Wayne that she gave on questioning was that he had not been able to tell his father about her marriage. [Written by Dr R.]

Discussion

1 Why does she find such difficulty telling her ex-husband about the marriage? Is she frightened about it?
2 The new husband is going to displace Wayne rather than the ex-husband. Is there more of a problem with Wayne than admitted? Why did she send him out? Did she say to Leonard what she came to say?

FOLLOW-UP FORM
Seminar No.69 (11.12.86)

Doctor: Dr L.

Patient: Wayne Denton & his mother

The new information :	Brought by mother for what she thought was a doctor-initiated follow-up, but doctor could not recall the request. Hearing, asthma, etc, all quiescent. Mother reported Wayne unable to tell father of mother's impending remarriage.
The forgotten information :	Only if follow-up actually requested.

1. *Had the doctor gained any new insight from :*

– *the previous surprise & consultation?*	Yes, in that the question of '*Who is the patient?*' has to be addressed continually
– *the previous presentation & discussion?*	No, from the last one, as the situation has seemed quiet.
Had this been used?	N/A
Was it useful?	N/A

2. *What connections did the patient make?*

	The possibility of Wayne being stressed by not being able to tell his father of his mother's impending marriage.
– *Did they engender surprise?*	Yes, in that it seemed to be Mrs D.'s business to tell rather than Wayne's.

3. *What connections did the doctor make :*

– *to the patient?*	None.
– *in presentation to the group?*	The displacement of responsibility from mother to son.

References to data

REFERENCES TO PATIENTS

Throughout this book twelve patients from our research discussions, conducted between 1984 and 1987, have been described to the reader. This has been done in such a way that some patients have been used on several occasions to illustrate quite different points about our research and way of working together. We have chosen this device because we were particularly interested in the fine detail of the cases we worked with. We list here the substitute names given to the patients which keep faith with how the doctor and the group referred to them. Thus some patients only have a first name and some only an initial letter while others have a title and surname. The following list shows at which seminars the patients were discussed:

	Patient	Seminar
1	Angela Denton & Wayne	9, 10, 16, 43, 61, 69
2	Ann Shipman	75, 76
3	Aurora	38, 43, 64
4	Mr F.	34
5	Jean Carter	46, 47
6	Mr Jennings	35, 40, 53, 70, 74, 81
7	Jill Norman	71
8	Lawrence B.	1, 3, 14
9	Mr & Mrs Miller	8, 18, 24, 30, 62
10	Sandra Morgan	71
11	Sharon	3, 6, 7, 16, 24, 40, 46, 58
12	Mrs Susan Towle	29, 31, 39, 59, 65, 67, 69

In the following list the patients are arranged by order of their appearance in the text showing the chapter number and the pages on which they appear.

Patient	Chapter	Page
Mr F.	1	4
Mrs Susan Towle	1	5, 6
	3	29–31
	7	76–9
Mrs Denton & Wayne	1	6, 7
	6	62–6
Jean Carter	1	7
	7	74–5
Lawrence B.	1	8–9
Mr Jennings	2	12–13, 15–17
	3	23–5
Sandra Morgan	3	26
	4	37
	6	66–8
Jill Norman	3	28–9
	6	68–9
Ann Shipman	3	31–2
	4	38
	5	56–9
Sharon	3	27–8
	4	39–43
Aurora	5	49–52
Mr & Mrs Miller	5	53–5

REFERENCES TO SEMINAR PARTICIPANTS

Mrs Balint speaks as E.B. and remains Enid when referred to in the discussion. The doctors have substitute names. They are given capital letters, prefixed by Dr, to indicate where they speak and corresponding first names when they refer to each other in the text of a discussion. So that they are either:

Dr B.	or	Brian
Dr D.	or	Dan
Dr G.	or	Gaby
Dr H.	or	Henry
Dr I.	or	Ian
Dr J.	or	Janet
Dr L.	or	Leonard
Dr N.	or	Nick
Dr O.	or	Oliver
Dr R.	or	Ruth

Bibliography

Bain, J. (1991) 'General Practices and the New Contract. II – Future Directions', *British Medical Journal* 302: 1247–9.

Balint, E. (1984) 'The History of Training and Research in Groups', *6th International Balint Conference*, Montreux.

Balint, E. and Norell, J. (eds) (1973) *Six Minutes for the Patient: Interactions in General Practice Consultations*, London: Tavistock.

Balint, M. (1957) *The Doctor, his Patient and the Illness*, revised 2nd edn, London: Pitman Paperbacks, 1968.

Bohr, N. (1933) 'Light and Life', Address delivered in 1932 to 11ème Congrès International de la Lumière, Copenhagen. *Nature* 131: 459.

Bohr, N. (1963) 'Light and Life Revisited', in Bohr, *Essays, 1958–1962, on Atomic Physics and Human Knowledge*, New York: Wiley-Interscience.

Britannica, 1988, Vol. 15, 159, Wallington, Surrey: Encyclopedia Britannica Ltd.

Brody, H. (1987) *Stories of Sickness*, New Haven, USA: Yale University Press.

Courtenay, M. (1968) *Sexual Discord in Marriage*, London: Tavistock.

Courtenay, M. and Hare, M. (1978) 'Difficult Doctors', *Journal of the Balint Society* 7: 14–19.

Elder, A. and Samuel, O. (eds) (1987) *While I'm Here, Doctor*, London: Tavistock.

Freeling, P. (1988) Book review of *While I'm Here, Doctor*, *British Medical Journal* 296: 1122.

Freud, S. *Papers on Techniques 1911–1915*. Standard Edition Vol. 12, Chapter 4, 114.

Gilley, J. (1988) 'Intimacy and Terminal Care', *Journal of the Royal College of General Practitioners* 38, 308: 121–2.

Harris, C. (1987) 'Let's Do Away With Counselling', *The Medical Annual: The Yearbook of General Practice*, Periera Gray, D.J. and Periera Gray, J. (eds), Bristol: Wright.

Harris, C. (1989) 'Seeing Sunflowers [William Pickles Lecture]', *Journal of the Royal College of General Practitioners* 39, 325: 313–19.

Howie, J.G.R. (1984) 'Research in General Practice: The Pursuit of Knowledge or the Defense of Wisdom', *British Medical Journal* 289: 1770–2.

Jenkins, R. and Shepherd, M. (1983) 'Mental Illness and General Practice', Chapter 7 in *Mental Illness; Changes and Trends*, Bean, P. (ed.), 15: 403–9, London: John Wiley & Sons.

Kuhn, T.S. (1970) *The Structure of Scientific Revolutions*, 2nd edn, Chicago: University of Chicago Press.

McWhinney, I.R. (1983) 'Changing Models: The Impact of Kuhn's Theory on Medicine', *Family Practice* 1, 1: 382.

Marinker, M. (1987) 'Journey to the Interior: The Search for Academic General Practice', *Journal of the Royal College of General Practitioners* 37, 302: 385–7.

Medawar, P.B. (1967) *The Art of the Soluble*, London: Pelican.

Medawar, P.B. (1969) *Induction and Intuition in Scientific Thought*, London: Methuen.

Nouwen, H. (1976) *Reaching Out*, London: William Collins, Fount Paperback Edition.

O'Dowd, T.C. (1988) 'Five Years of Heartsick Patients in General Practice', *British Medical Journal* 297: 528–30.

Pellegrino, E.D. (1979) In Englehardt, H.I. *et al.* (eds) *Clinical Judgement: A Critical Approach*, Holland: Reidel.

Pendleton, D. and Haslet, J. (eds) (1983) *Doctor–Patient Communication*, London: Academic Press.

Pendleton, D. *et al.* (1984) *The Consultation: An Approach to Learning and Teaching*, Oxford General Practice Series, Oxford: OUP.

Polanyi, M. (1958) *Personal Knowledge: Towards a Post-Critical Philosophy*, London: Routledge & Kegan Paul.

Popper, K.R. (1963) *Conjectures and Refutations*, London: Routledge & Kegan Paul.

Rosenfeld, L. (1963) 'Niels Bohr's Contribution to Epistemology', *Physics Today* 16: 10.

Rowland, N., Irving, J. and Maynard, A. (1989) 'Can General Practitioners Counsel?', *Journal of the Royal College of General Practitioners* 39, 320: 118.

Salinsky, J. (1989) 'Do We Still Need an Analyst for a Leader?', *Journal of the Balint Society* 17: 33.

Whewell, W. (1840) *The Philosophy of the Inductive Sciences*, London: John Parker.

Winnicott, D. (1972) 'Discussion at a Meeting of the British Psychoanalytic Society in 1940'. Recorded in *The Theory of the Parent Infant Relationship*, London: Hogarth Press.

Index